About a Cabbage

ANDREW KINGSTON

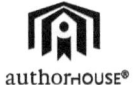

authorHOUSE®

AuthorHouse™ UK Ltd.
500 Avebury Boulevard
Central Milton Keynes, MK9 2BE
www.authorhouse.co.uk
Phone: 08001974150

First published by AuthorHouse 2/5/2010

ISBN: 978-1-4490-7392-3 (sc)

This book is printed on acid-free paper.

Introduction

I am a 54 years old white man, twenty three stone in weight, six feet three inches tall and running to fat, I have three chins and counting.

I am very heterosexual; I am not at all confused about that, I am intelligent and rather unreasonably opinionated.

I know nor care nothing for politics, religion or ethnic issues though am always ready to defend my miss informed corner with my share of bigoted, racist piousness, my God being bigger than yours sort of thing.

I know that there is a God, I am also aware that he / she doesn't like me an awful lot as when they say "shit happens" it happens to me far too often.

I have an opinion on everything, it is important to have an opinion even if it is wrong or even offensive, a no comment to me means you were not listening to the question.

I am a confirmed petrol head with a liking for good cars and fast motor bikes and it is my blessing that I have had quite a few of both, I have averaged forty thousand plus miles per year for the past thirty years and consider myself to be fast but safe, I enjoy the risk but have had few crashes or accidents off of the race track and my license, although endorsed many times in nearly forty years of motoring, has at the moment only two endorsements.

I look young for my age, have never looked like I am ill and always appear to be smiling, probably badly fitting false teeth, I am young at heart bordering on immature which my contemporaries and life partners find rather annoying.

My partner spends a lot of time apologising for things that I have said or done though we always get invited back, I always make people laugh, I am a clown and life is my circus.

The first thing that I did when I found out that I was very ill was to go out and buy a rather expensive motorbike, it is not my intention to die in a bed, my biggest fear being someone wiping my arse with long finger nails.

The only time that I feel really alive is when I am scaring myself silly on a bike, either on the road or a circuit, speed and danger are the most fantastic of all drugs, fear can be completely free and is not really addictive.

I have taken this opportunity to sit and write this story about the changes to my life, changes that have given me the time to become fat, opinionated and rather broad in the arse department, sat around with nothing better to do with my time, if I am not seen to be busy my partner will always find something for me to do, so I am doing this, to look busy as I am not fond of ironing.

I have never in my life lived alone so have never had to make a bed, do any ironing, hoover or dust etc, that is until now.

I do it now because some clown wrote in the leaflet that I received when I left the hospital, that these tasks are good exercise and therapeutic, I could strangle the bitch because I now have to make the bed and do some selective ironing and be very therapeutic…

I have had quite a good life really, I have been to an awful lot of places and done an awful amount of awful things with awful people and I am not at all surprised as to how I find myself now, pleasantly awful.

I have abused myself beyond reason, risked all for little more than fun, taken my place among the fools of this world and made folly a bi word.

I will try and explain to you why I am covered in scars.

I am English, born into a military family in North London which is where my family roots are, my father being a soldier in the Royal Horse Guards though I doubt he ever sat a horse in his life.

Being a tall good looking man with a film star cleft chin he would have fitted the part rather well I think and often think of him whenever they troop the colour or change the guard, often with a tear in my eye, I have always missed him so much.

The regiment was a tank regiment, predominately armoured cars of various makes, Alvis built Saladin's, Saracens' and the smaller Ferrets, hit and run style missions, recognisance, that sort of thing, though he never fought in a true war, he did go to both Aden and Cyprus as part of peace keeping forces, and long tours of duty in Western Europe though I was robbed of the chance to have the conversations with him.

My father was a self educated man who specialised in radio and radar when it was very very basic stuff and up until his early and un timely death at the age of thirty seven, was a happy man with his lot, doing something as a job that really interested him, he even did it when he came home and built from scratch his own equipment.

I still remember his radio call sign, G3RRZ George three Roger Roger Zulu and would often hear him talking to someone on the other side of the world on a radio that he had knocked up out of spare bits and bobs, the smell of solder lingering in the air.

He became ill quite suddenly with a heart attack while out on exercise and never recovered dying the following year during an attempt to repair his heart, he died on the operating table, I never got to say the things that I have wanted to say for forty years now.

He was buried with a full military funeral, many of his contemporaries in attendance and it was all too much for us children, the whole scene too big for our little minds and huge scars were burnt into me, never to be erased.

As children we were introduced to various stations throughout the world living for a number of years in Germany and in Cyprus, happy times all,

with good exposure to alternative cultures, different climates, dangerous circumstances, unreasonable behaviour from what seems unreasonable people but excellent exposure for any child none the less even if at times we were exposed to a mini war zone.

My mother was also from London's east end, daughter of a tailor and always a loving and popular woman, a good mother and friend, excellent dancer and swimmer, always singing while doing her daily chores.

Following my fathers death she became both mum and dad to us, my four siblings and I, able to love and discipline in equal measure although barely five feet tall, something that has not changed over the years and we all love her dearly, I still think she looks just like our Queen though.

She has been fortunate to re marry, a local man from the end of the road that we grew up in, in Windsor, Berkshire, following my fathers demise.

He has always been a lovely man, never trying to replace my father, always a friend to guide me, help me, care for me.

It was after my father had died from heart disease that we, collectively, were made aware of our genetic make up, that nearly all males from my paternal side had died of heart related problems and usually died very early in their lives or at best had surgery and a life time of care and medication.

We had been protected from this information till now, our globe trotting life style had excluded us from our immediate families and the fate of the clan was news to us, in fact up until this point I was not even aware that we had a clan, a gene belt so to speak as I do not recall ever meeting a grand father, uncles or other except from my mothers side who have the habit of hanging on for ages.

It was presumed that my brothers and I, Tony, Stuart and Mark would indeed suffer the same fate, not an unreasonable assumption as we will later see and I have spent all of my adult years waiting to die and as such no risk was too great, anything was ok and I have had a huge amount of injuries and surgery pursuing this foolish policy, but had I not pursued this policy I may well be saying if only I had done this and if only I had done that, instead I did it reasoning that this might be my demise, but what a demise when compared to dying in a hospital bed.

My mother had once said to me "If you have half of your fathers courage, you will be a man" and I have strived for that recognition all of my life, never feeling as though I had achieved it.

My elder brother Tony was clearly from my mother's side of the family, fair and slender, healthy and athletic having at times competed for the RAF in track events, and I have excluded my sister also for this reason.

My younger brothers Stuart and Mark were like me, following more in our fathers foot steps, I am by far the largest and obviously the most at risk because I look very much like my father though my brother Stuart was the first to need some attention for heart related issues other than blood pressure tablets which I think we were both on from quite an early age.

Life progressed for me through three failed marriages and five children to where I now find myself, not a very good place.

I have gone from wealth to broke, had it all to having nothing, very happy to completely and utterly miserable.

I have had many adventures throughout the world, climbing, skiing, sailing, racing cars and motor bikes, in fact I could say that I have done it and bought the tee shirt though given more time I am quite sure that there are lots of silly things that I haven't tried yet.

I have been in more punch ups than I care to remember, fought men who I shouldn't have, winning and losing in equal measure though facially managed to remain largely unmarked apart from scars to both eyelids and eyebrows and quite a few teeth missing.

I have endured many injuries, broken both elbows, both ankles, some toes, a few fingers, both thumbs, most of my teeth, my nose, my left collar bone and my right leg to say the least.

I remember a rather difficult fortnight when I fell twisting my ankle till it broke, as I went over I ruptured my cruciate ligament in my knee and that same week while watering the garden with a plaster cast on both legs the handle came off of the watering can, the full can dropping onto my foot breaking my big toe, oh joy..

I have had some forty operations including surgery on my cock and my tonsils, both of my knees, both arms, my eyes and on my back.

I have managed to lose an eye, lose my virginity and very much lose my way.

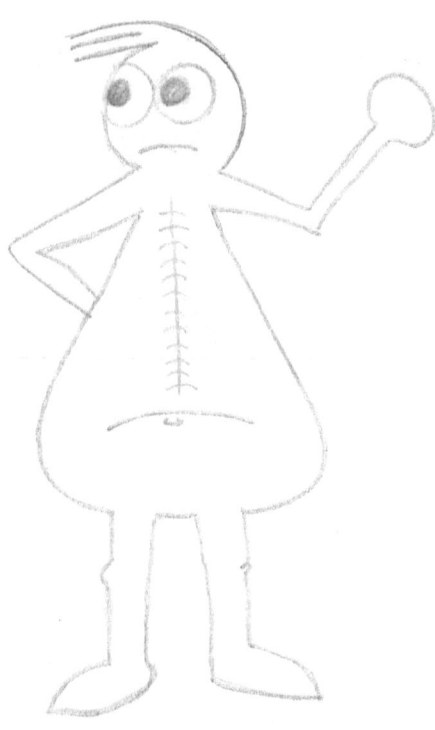

Chapter one

At school I always managed to please my mother by getting an A for every lesson except sport or physical education, at which I was utter crap, my feet seemed to belong to a stranger never doing what I wanted of them and always tripping me up, I did however become a champion at picking up bean bags with my toes, it was supposed to strengthen my legs ?

I was very interested in a God so even managed to do well in religious studies, most unusual at my school as this lesson was normally just a good skive with the teachers having a rather difficult time selling the product to children who had not been raised Christians, not heathens, just not Christians.

I had a bent towards the sciences, what, when and why being what made me tick and was a high achiever at art being able to draw and paint very well though never able to please the master because I was often away with the fairies, doodling or painting what I thought and not the subject matter as instructed.

I have always taken things apart, from a tiny watch to a huge V8 motor engine and have now an extensive knowledge of how things work, my motor bikes, from a very early age, being constantly in bits and improvements always on the drawing board, finances willing. On occasion I could also put things back together again, not always sadly.

Anything mechanical interests me, I can see beauty in a piece of metal and I find steam power incredibly emotional and interesting and fully understand the dream of driving a steam engine, train spotters on the other hand are a really sad bunch of twats.

My main subject ended up being mathematics, I had developed a massive ability to recall, I could remember information, carry out all manner of calculations in my head and even today find myself multiplying peoples number plates to stave of boredom while sat in traffic.

I am however not a geek nor a dork, I am barely computer literate and frequently press the wrong key setting off a rage or tantrum as I struggle to find out what I have done wrong, again and frequently having to pay a real geek to come and put it right for me.

I got my first motor vehicle on my sixteenth birthday, a beautiful Vespa 180ss scooter, bright blue and chrome and I managed to fall off of it within ten minutes starting a life time of accidents with vehicles, though to be fair, I was attempting my first ever wheelie, hoisting the front wheel up in the air before I had learnt how to keep it down on the Tarmac.

The scooter opened up a whole new world of opportunity, the girls liked transport and in those days there was no crash helmet law so any one could just jump on the back of the scooter and off we would go, it got me laid an awful lot of times and I was to have several other scooters while in my teens and many an adventure.

Recalling the trips down to Cornwall each year with my school mates, we had all finished school by now but remained a loyal little group for a couple of years until life's opportunities took us all in different directions.

We would always manage to choose the weeks that it would piss down with rain and we would always be camping. One of our group discovered that if you cut the closed corners off of a dustbin bag and another hole for your head it was possible to make water proof waist coats which kept most of him warm and dry, we all quickly copied him.

I remember the time that I managed to get the girl from the café at Perrinporth beach onto the back of my scooter, giving her a lift home from work with a promise to collect her later to go on a date.

She looked fabulous and we scooted into the local town and met up with all of my mates, Andy, Andy, Sean and Paul, there were three called Andy in our group of five, and they all had a girl in tow from the café or beach shop.

We danced and had a really good fun evening taking the girls home on our scooters when the club closed, we were all sixteen so it was a teens club and no drink was served, I use the word club quite loosely as well because it was a village hall with most of the bulbs taken out of the lamps and a few flashing disco lights working in time with the frantic music.

When we got close to this girls house, she will remain nameless except in my heart, she said "pull over hear" and I pulled in to pull into a small gated road and she started to kiss me.

I had no sooner got my blood up when she jumped off the scooter and ran for it yelling "goodbye" and "sorry", sorry for what I was thinking as all hell let loose.

Her dad was walking his sheep dog down the lane and had decided, seeing my intentions with his daughter, to give me both barrels, at an extreme range I must admit, but some of it bounced off me anyway, scaring the living daylights out of me, obviously he had seen her run for it first.

It is funny how your machine never starts first go when you really need it too, I dined out on this story for ages, but cleaned the spark plug and the carburettor for good measure the very next day, just in case.

My working career has been both varied and quite interesting never really staying at anything too long and I have included a snippet or two to add some flavour to my character references.

My first job was as a Saturday boy in the local fish mongers, my mum being a regular client had asked the boss if he needed a weekend lad and as I had just turned fourteen, he took me on.

It was an old established shop with old established fresh fish and poultry methods, none of this new fangled, pre packaged stuff.

The fresh fish was always collected from billingsgate market in London every morning at five o'clock and would then be displayed on a huge wet slab, wet because of the gigantic block of ice at its head that dribbled ice cold water down the sloping slab throughout the day as it slowly melted away, never, not even in the heat of summer, did it melt away completely though.

The boss, Norman, was a huge great bear of a man who judged my manhood on my ability to carry this block of ice from the truck outside and into and onto the slab, something that he could easily do by resting it on his rather rotund belly, I couldn't do it because I had yet to develop the belly and it would slip from my grasp, but I was working on it. He would say "you'll be a proper man when you can carry that lad".

There could be as many as twenty different species of fish from cod through haddock, sole and plaice, herring and mackerel as well as smoked fish.

There was always a good stock of squid, shell fish and live crab and lobster for those that could afford it.

The other side of the shop was for poultry and game ranging from the humble chicken through all manner of water foul and ending up with some wonderful hare, venison and rabbit hanging from the ceiling on hooks.

I was treated really well by the other shop staff, the shop owner and best of all by the shop owner's wife who introduced me to all things sex, as soon as I was nearly sixteen. I had also taken up motorcycling and it was quite funny learning to ride all of these things all at once, only one had handle bars though.

It was in these formative years that I learnt how to hold and use tools, learnt the trade of the fish mongers when all the fish were whole and fresh, cold and slimy, not ready filleted and frozen, some even being alive pending despatch, death by boiling water.

The smoked fish was salted and coloured in a bath of dye and then smoked to varying degrees depending on the end product but all done in house, something that just doesn't happen anymore, beautiful oak smoked fish, as much as eight to eighteen hours in the making, really professional and very satisfying.

I would normally grab a piece of fish or shell fish and warm it through in a pan for my breakfast every morning, a huge chunk of fresh bread from the bakers next door and a mug of tea and sometimes I would even remember to wash my hands first..........

In the bakers shop next door was a really lovely girl, Elizabeth, who I had been eying up for quite some time.

She never had a boyfriend, never was seen out and about even though she really was quite beautiful and I decided to make an even bigger effort to befriend her, saw her several times a day just to chat and buy even more scones, bread etc.

Eventually she gave in and we went out in my newly acquired first car, a mini 850cc in British racing green and wood interior, really smart, though terribly underpowered, I was two weeks into my seventeenth year.

We went to a dance, a bar and then I took her home by eleven as promised to her Dad.

Her parents were not at home and we settled down in the garden on a swing chair for a kiss and a cuddle, she really was lovely.

All of a sudden and with no warning she started to look strange and fell onto the floor shaking and shuddering from head to foot, foaming at the mouth and I was bloody terrified.

Her mum and dad had just got home and heard me yelling, came into the garden and took control of the situation, her father leading me away with her mother comforting Elizabeth.

Her father explained to me that his daughter suffered from epilepsy, not a lot could be done about it in those days and that they would prefer if I left, I did.

Elizabeth couldn't face me again, left her job in the bakers and I never set eyes on her again, I did however manage to shed a few pounds in weight now that I didn't have to eat all of those scones and dough nuts.

This was a good time for me, I was mobile and could drive the company Transit pick up truck, not only to the market but out and about doing deliveries, the restaurants, the posh houses and best of all, Windsor safari park had about a quarter of a tonne of fish every day for the seals, sea lions and the huge great Orca, the killer whale.

The trainer, John Savage, was quite fearless with the Orca, he would get into the water and play with it, I would look on terrified for him and always waited for that fateful day when something would go wrong, I was there when it did.

John was standing on the edge of the pool feeding the Orca fresh mackerel, which the whale really did appear to enjoy, when the whale closed its mouth around Johns hand and started to sink below the water taking him with it. The viewing area was always closed at feeding time because of this risky business of feeding mixed with training sessions.

John called out for help just before he sunk below the surface and I was the only person around, help, what did he mean help, what the hell was I supposed to do, I am not scared of much but this killer whale, the clue is in its name, was on my very scared of list along with other things that bite and sting.

Luckily it was all over as quickly as it began, John had another fish in his other hand and he waved it in front of the whale's eye and the whale let him go to get at the fish, mackerel was after all his favourite tipple and he was only playing, in a drowning you sort of way.

John at no time blamed the whale for his broken hand, he still spoke to the whale very calmly before he was taken off to A&E to get his hand fixed up and he was away from the pool for a month though always in the background, he loved his whale.

The above had a profound effect on me, I couldn't bring myself to get into a public swimming pool let alone go into the sea for an awful long time and still fear being out of my depth.

I loved this period of my life, although never overpaid; I was comfortable, enjoyed my work and my social life and was moving forward, though at times just couldn't get the smell off of my hands when I was going out.

At festive periods all of the staff from the shop, old Jack excluded because he was just very old, would travel to local farms to get the poultry, not frozen as is normal today, all still walking and feathered, noisy and smelling quite foul, yes I know, excuse the pun.

I was to learn how to catch, kill, pluck and dress all manner of bird from huge thirty pound turkeys through to tiny grouse and everything in between.

I was taught how to skin and dress hare, rabbit and venison to name but a few and I did it all with immense pride, no waste meat left anywhere and all offal bagged up ready for making the gravy.

I also learned how to bleed as I would cut myself frequently and quite often bad enough to need stitching up at the local hospital, there was no such thing as an armoured glove in those days.

Some of the worst injuries came from drawing out the guts of animals that had been shot, the gun shots breaking their ribs and forcing bits of bone through the abdomen, readily cutting probing digits.

It is a very gut turning experience to be drawing out the innards of game birds or hare that have been hung up to mature for a week, the blow fly maggots crawling all over your hands and up your arm, it really took some getting used to.

I worked in the fish mongers up till I was eighteen and ready to go to work at the ICI paint factory in Slough, Berkshire where I had designs on joining the company fire brigade, which I did six weeks after setting foot on the site.

The in house fire brigade was one of make do and mend, the main task being to show willing and attend to minor incidents or at best delaying tactics pending the arrival of the county brigade and accordingly the vehicles and appliances were very much second best and cheap.

This was quite a worry when you consider that ICI Slough is surrounded with houses, schools etc and if it were to go up in flames, several thousand people would be ever so slightly pissed off and possibly or probably very much at risk.

I would have to attend weekly practise sessions which were always a good laugh, two hours spent setting up all of the gear to spend thirty seconds extinguishing a bucket of diesel that was more risk from the smoke than the flame, but I really didn't like the ladder work and no amount of reminding the leader that I was driving the engine and couldn't get up the ladder and operate the pumps so why did I have to bother, would get me out of it.

There were two main fire engines at the small sit fire station, the first being a twenty five year old green goddess Bedford ex RAF fire tender which seemed to be in the most wonderful condition and was utterly reliable, the other, the one that I was to drive, was a very old series Landrover which again in good condition was actually a complete monster of a vehicle and quite unsuitable for the task set before it.

It had a crash gearbox with no synchronising of the gears what so ever, and it was so under powered that if it was full of water, two hundred gallons, it would take so long to gain speed, accelerate being a big word for it, that it would slow down too much while you tried to get it to change gear and you would have to stop and start again.

Add to this the very restricted steering lock which meant that it had to do three point turns on junctions that articulated lorries could get round and no power steering, no power on the brakes etc you will start to get the picture.

All this awful driving would be happening while three men in the back would be trying to get into their respective fire fighting suits and breathing equipment, cursing the crashing of the gearbox and the swearing at me pulling and pushing on the steering and swinging from side to side wobbling its way through the very busy built up site trying desperately not to run anyone over while pumping the over loaded rotten brakes.

If this vehicle ever had to attend a true first shout at a true fire I do believe the problem would burn itself out long before I arrived on the scene.

My actual job was making the bases for all ICI paint products which involved the blending of solvents, pigments and varnishes in differing recipes using different kinds of machines and I very badly twisted a knee one evening requiring surgery to unlock the ruptured cartilage and quite a long time off of work.

Once back to work it was discovered that I could no longer run, couldn't be in the fire service and I decided to leave the job as it was also interfering with my courting young ladies.

I went to work for Slough council on a black gang, a tarmac crew, highway repairs and small works.

In those days, patching and maintenance to the highways, along with dropped crossings, traffic light installation etc was undertaken in house, council employees did the work and I really enjoyed the work, hard but quite well paid and in the summer, most agreeable to me though I didn't stay too long, though I did spend a period at college learning how to cut stone, I didn't know at the time that this would be a skill I would not use again for more than ten years. I had become very fit and strong with quite a nice tan by working out doors all day in all weathers.

It was while cutting a kerb using a pneumatic breaker that I was hit very hard in the face by a piece of concrete which unfortunately damaged my sight, removing the retina from the back of my left eye requiring extensive surgery, this being the days before laser surgery, they cut their way through the front of the eye, did what they had to do, and sewed it all back together again, yuck.

I was to remove this retina a further three times before it was to knackered to go back on and although is attached, is so corrugated that it is next to useless and I am blind in my left eye.

I always recall the day that my younger sister Sally paid me a visit in the eye ward, I couldn't see her coming though was sure it was her because of the noise her shoes made.

When she got by my bed, I turned to face her when she called my name and on seeing my face she passed out and was carted off to A&E to make sure that she was ok, she didn't come to see me after all, my face was black and blue with two strawberry coloured eyes and I looked satanic.

I have just taken a job in the local slaughter house today as the money was better and I have moved in to a flat with my new girl friend and need the extra money. The worst thing here was the terrible smell, it could get so bad that at times it felt like it could burn the skin from the inside of your nose and if you tried to breath through your mouth, the taste was worse than the smell.

I seem to have spent a lot of my early life killing things, a bit of a worry, it could become a habit.

My initiation here was to be thrown into a huge tank full of warm pigs blood which was destined to be turned into black pudding, I hope I didn't change the flavour too much, I wasn't in it that long.

It would seem that a cow was to revenge my dipping as the very next day a hefty great cow that I had just put a bolt in its head, decided to get up again and make a run for it taking the shift foreman by the leg and carrying him on one horn out of the building into the car park before it realised that it was supposed to be dead and succumbed to its injuries, the foreman survived.

This place was to close down, a casualty of frozen or imported meats which along with the frozen fish was decimating these wonderful old trades.

I then worked air side at Heathrow airport loading aircraft but I couldn't stand the theft that was going on from peoples luggage and was forced to leave by my conscience, no wonder it was then called thief row and I moved to driving lorries throughout the south of England for the next few years, something that I really did enjoy and which gave me an enviable knowledge of London and the home counties.

I was by now in my mid twenties and rather well built, delivering huge bales of cloth to sweat shops throughout London's east end, I was now twenty stone and as fit as a butchers dog.

My best friend in the whole world was my partner in crime here, it was mostly a two man job so the vehicles had two man crews and Doug Hayes and I had a really good time, really enjoyed going to work.

I was later, when I was coming up for thirty two, to get a job as service manager of a Fiat dealership in Henley on Thames, I think more for my enthusiasm for the post rather than any previous knowledge of running a busy workshop though in fairness I did have a huge knowledge of vehicles and was very good at maths so learning the minor details was rather easy for me.

This job lasted for a year or so before the garage closing down, the owner being a drunk had spent all of the profit. The main benefit from this employment was a company car, my first and something that I found increasingly important as time went on.

It was also my first proper job at managing staff and running someone else's business, something that I did not truly enjoy, all of the work, none of the money.

I next moved into mobile crane driving, working on construction sites throughout the south of England, mainly home counties and found this, once my training was out of the way and I had a plant operator's license, very agreeable.

It completely satisfied my fascination for all things mechanical, huge monster size vehicles sometimes with up to nine axles, all wheel drives, all wheel steering, off road and on, always something interesting going on.

I could sit in my crane when on site watching and learning skills that were being acted out in front of me and I vowed that one day I would start my very own construction company which I very soon did, due to a down turn in the building industries which put us plant operators onto a three day week, not enough money to pay my mortgage or feed the kids.

I bought a small Leyland van which my children named Bert, I advertised in the local papers and was instantly busy all over the county and growing with every passing day.

Four companies later, I am still doing it having lost a business each and every time that I have divorced, bloody woman always win especially if there are kids involved.

I have been quite well off and then have sod all more times than I want to remember, driving a Mercedes one week and a Ford the next, small flat one month and big house the next all dependant on where I stand in a marriage.

Although I am far from unique, I do not understand women, I really haven't got a clue when they whine at me, huffing and puffing that I do not care for them, do not listen to them or take any notice of them, they are of course utterly correct, I have never heard a woman say anything interesting yet, and I do not go in for emotional blackmail, I completely refuse to grovel around trying to make a relationship work, if it isn't working, I just give up and normally leave.

Why o why will a woman not just tell you what is the matter so that if you want to you can do something about it, take away the guessing, please.

I have taken four weeks off work to have my tonsils out, I keep getting throat infections and have been on all sorts of medication for more than ten years, none of which now helps so the consultant has decided that although I am rather old for this, being forty two now, he feels it to be the only way forward.

I duly attend the Oxford Infirmary, now closed and gone, and have my operation, the surgeon being perfectly correct when he told me that I was in for a rough time, you would have thought I had had my testicles removed it was so painful.

I couldn't stop bleeding and spent two weeks sat up in bed pending whether they were going to operate again but in the end all was well.

The worse part of the whole procedure is being forced to eat toast and cornflakes for breakfast and lunch, to remove the muck from the back of my throat, it could have been glass and wood shavings it hurt so much.

The above procedure also changed my voice, I have always been a good singer, now it is more of a croaker than a crooner

Chapter two

I met my current and I might add final partner on an internet site, she lived just eight miles away and following e-mail exchanges and conversations we agreed to meet up.

I was my usual self, worked too late and arrived just as she was about to leave our pre arranged destination in the centre of Thame, just outside of Oxford.

Linda is slight of stature, quiet, kind and thoughtful of person, attractive for a grandmother and always great fun to be with.

We had a really good evening, we both fell head over heals that first night and have been together for three years now and I have been added to her list of possessions, that's what I feel, I am not me, I am part of her, an extension of her.

If this fails to work out I will most definitely live alone because I now find the whole giving thing annoying, soaps on TV, holidays when it is not convenient, meat and three veg every night, clearing up all of the time and clutter, why cover every surface with clutter and then complain that everything is covered in dust, why not stop buying clutter......

Just after I had met Linda, I had a check up with a new doctor who called me on my mobile shortly after our appointment and requested that I went to see her again as she now had the results back from the lab.

She advised me that I had very high blood pressure, my cholesterol was off the scale and that I had become diabetic, wow, all in one go.

I started drugs for the blood pressure as well as ulcer busting drugs because they had already discovered that I had one, and also started to take tablets for the newly diagnosed diabetes.

I was issued with a small machine to check my blood sugar, I had to prick myself and then let the machine measure the sugar levels and I could adjust my drugs or diet accordingly to stay within a pre determined value, what a palaver

My youngest children were very keen to help me do it though, always getting the machine out and pricking my fingers far more times than was really needed but it amused them, for a while.

This was in the march of 2006 and Linda and I planned a holiday in Egypt for late October into early November which we duly went on and had quite a good time, not good enough to want to return there again though.

Shamil Sheik is a dirty shit hole, built up to take advantage of the tourist trade that this red Sea area fully deserves but it stinks of sewage and rotting rubbish, not the sea which is beautiful, I mean the streets though non of it was as bad as Cairo which has rubbish stacked up in the streets.

We were sat in the most wonderful of settings in a restaurant beside the Nile, I could dangle my fingers in the water while sat at the table and floating down the Nile river past me would be tons and tons of rubbish, no one picked anything up, just dropped it on the floor.

The people that we met were lying, robbing, two faced Arabs who take our shilling but actually despise us for our relationship with the US and associations with Israel, they consider that they are still at war, no declaration of peace has ever been reached and nearly all Egyptians will at some time or another serve in the Army or police forces.

The military are everywhere, road blocks and checks every few miles, no go areas and a general air of hostility, it is always wise to have a guide, one who can also speak some English and bribes are a way of life, that's not to say that they do not come across as friendly, they do, it is just not what they really think of us.

It is also very unfortunate that nearly all of the good diving sites are outside of the resort so we were forced to travel to these less than friendly areas, hey ho, I only wanted to go somewhere where it is warm, didn't want all of the political shit that goes with it, they would however, do well to clean up their act as well as their rubbish if the country intends to prosper from tourism , though they are not unique, it is like this throughout Africa.

During the holiday I became increasingly tired, something that we put down to the heat, the food and the shits that I always succumb to when ever I go abroad though we still managed to go snorkelling, camel trekking in the desert and swimming in the sea near our resort, wandering around to different restaurant every evening and the most enduring memory is of Linda falling out of a hammock, she did hurt herself though, sorry for laughing so much but it really was very funny to watch especially given the amount of time it took you to get into it in the first place.

I did however spend quite some time just floating around giving all of the wonderful fish names, thin ones associated to thin people that I know etc this did make Linda laugh. I would say "did you see that David that just swam by"

We even visited the famous pyramids, rearing up out of the sand in the suburbs of Cairo, which were crap I might add as I have had more interesting building sites which didn't have people trying to mug you every ten minutes, sorry, ten seconds, even the police stand in your way when taking a photo then hold their hand out for money, getting out a camera is a sure way to get a crowd around you.

We didn't bother queuing up to take a tour inside the pyramid because I wasn't up to it and it would have just been another excuse to be mugged, even the famous sphinx was more like a concrete pussy cat, terribly disappointing after the journey to get there, they always seem to make these things look so grand and big on the TV, one should never meet their heroes

I was lucky, when back in England, to watch a program on the TV where Ewan McGregor and Charlie Boreman visited Cairo and they were allowed to take a camera crew into the pyramid with them so I got to see what it was like inside without the journey, a journey that I now know I would not have been able to complete.

We journeyed into central Cairo and following lunch, Linda had a good look around the very famous and very good museum of ancient antiquities, lots of mummies and stuff.

I couldn't manage to stand up any longer, my legs were swelling and I didn't know why, I do now.

We had to spend quite a lot of time just lounging around the pool at our hotel, not the best hotel I have ever stayed at, in fact I wish I had paid a lot more for our holiday but as this was my first time here I was not to know that three start means shite, shite food, shite pool and shite entertainment.

I just couldn't get well enough for anything else but lazing around, fortunately Linda and I both had unfinished books and it was quite hot so was nice to have a swim and a drink every half an hour or so, Linda always moving her pool chair to stay in the sun, me always moving mine to stay out of it, it must have looked like we had had a falling out, we were seldom close together.

On our return to the UK I had to go to Aylesbury hospital for a chat with a knee consultant as both of my knees have now succumbed to abuse and failed, mind you, they have both endured five surgical procedures over the years so it is about time to replace them with some nice shiny steel ones.

During the blood tests, why do they always have to take blood, I passed out and the nursing staff diagnosed me as being a woos, upset by the sight of blood etc but carted me unconscious down to the accident and emergency department where I was checked out with an ECG and a rather rushed examination.

The nurses had barely got a needle into my arm when the very busy doctor proclaimed that I was free to go, he had just managed to be the first of many who rushed me through and got it wrong, I had just had a heart attack and though it didn't show on his ECG was to come up as a scar later when this test was repeated by someone a little more talented and a little bit more thorough.

I have often wondered how many people have died as a result of this doctors rushing around and while I can appreciate his being busy, I find his end results somewhat dangerous.

The doctor, bless him, announced that I was a woos, a delicate little flower, and had in fact fainted at the site of blood and I was dismissed to go home, I was feeling very embarrassed for wasting his and the nursing staff's valuable time because I believed him as well which is a bit daft thinking about the amount of blood that I had seen over the years in the fish mongers and later in the abattoirs, and that's without the amount of my own liquid contents that I had spilt.

On arriving home I was feeling decidedly delicate, a feeling of unwell and quite light headed with a nasty aching feeling in my left shoulder and arm.

I had my tea and spent a restless night with this continuing ache and unrest, not being able to get comfortable or settled and I kept Linda awake as well which is asking for trouble.

I went off to work the following morning, I favour early starts because of the traffic free roads and always travel to my furthest point first so that my journey home is the shortest and therefore quickest.

I had just got a brand new car, and really enjoyed driving it, little did I know that I would not be doing it for four months to come.

I recalled at this time that my previous doctor had been injecting steroids into my left shoulder when I had complained of this constant aching and it turned out to be the start of heart problems and not a frozen shoulder as diagnosed.

I was thinking little about what had happened the previous day and after a few meetings, a few site visits I pottered off towards home and the end of day paperwork, e-mails and phone messages, I was at this time still in the building trade, general manager of my own company.

My hands, more the left side, was feeling rather numb, my fingers seemed as though they were all joined together, webbed, stiff and I recognised that I had been feeling this on and off for quite a few months and had been putting it down to age, rheumatism even.

I ate my evening meal and had my usual cigarette on the terrace and sat down to watch the TV with Linda when it all started to go wrong, my world came crashing in on me.

I had this feeling of not being able to get my breath and the ache was right down my left arm and up into my jaw, my fingers were stiff, I couldn't move them independently of each other again and speaking had now become difficult. It was just like being very very pissed.

Linda could see that I was really in trouble as I collapsed into her arms, her terrified with what confronted us, me apologising as best I could, and us both in tears, me saying goodbye and her being so brave and telling me everything would be just fine. As I started to pass out again I recall saying "I have to go now" to which Linda replied " Go where love" which made me smile, I was quite sure that I was dying, I could see the light down the tunnel.

I was too scared to speak, even had I been able to, Linda called an ambulance and not for the first time the fire engine turned up, they carried a paramedic and were much closer than either ambulance station, Oxford or Aylesbury though I did wonder if you would get an ambulance if you requested a fire engine.

The paramedic and his crew of fire fighters were very good, gave me oxygen and packaged me up ready for the ambulance which was outside within ten minutes, making notes and getting information from Linda, all terribly professional, polished even, instilling calm in a situation where I wanted to scream, comfort and safety when needed most.

Between them all they managed to stretcher me out to the ambulance, getting past the cars and across the front lawn let alone down the three nasty little steps, steps that have caught a lot of people out because they can be very difficult to see. I remember the site of my rather large eldest daughter as she turned to wave goodbye and missing the first of the steps, falling full tilt flat on her front, but because her front bumps are so massive she didn't hit her face on the ground and it looked like someone had

abandoned a wheel barrow on the path. It was quite impossible for me to help her up, she had started to cry and that just made things worse because I was in fits of laughter, seldom have I seen anything so funny.

I was administered anti vomit medicines and some morphine via the needle which had been swiftly stuck in my arm and taped into place and after a few minutes off we all went to the hospital in Aylesbury, Buckinghamshire, Linda following behind in her little car, sirens and blue lights doing their thing as we raced along, only ten miles to the hospital.

Sadly the doctor who had sent me on my way the previous day was not on duty so I had to recall what had gone on and was, following more tests dumped in a side area pending transportation to a hospital 10 miles away in High Wycombe, Bucks where they had the facility to look into heart related problems, and this is where the fun really begins, it was a really scary time for me, this was not unexpected but that didn't reduce the intensity of the situation that I now find myself in, scared, worried and wishing for my mum.

My brother Stuart popped into see me, I wish the arsehole hadn't because all he could complain about was the business, the vehicles, him, him, him.

He didn't mention me once, not once and we parted company like we usually do, with bad feelings.

Note, my brother was supposed to be looking after my / our business while I was ill and incapacitated.

Chapter three

The High Wycombe general hospital could manage to carry out cardiac investigations using a catheter which allowed them to look into and around your heart in real time, and I had, four days later, an Angio gram.

It was very strange to walk down to the catheter laboratory where these procedures are carried out, wearing only a gown and my slippers, I did in fact have another gown on backwards to cover my bottom as the gowns are one size fits all but fit no one, but no underwear what so ever, difficult to sit down and keep your legs shut when you are a bloke so I had to stand while waiting my turn which makes my legs ache, hey ho, I knew it was going to be an awful day because I had to wait for so long that I was really rough by the time I was seen.

Once in the lab you are laid out on a very distinctive table, shaped like a body and surrounded with electronic equipment and screens as well as at least a dozen people. Your name is checked and a needle inserted into the back of your hand, just in case you need anything, this worried me a bit, like what could I possibly need that could be pushed through that little hole.

Once settled and naked, but for a blanket, you have your groin washed and shaved and a small incision is made in the right hand groin, a catheter is inserted into the femal artery (right next to my goolies) and a wire, for want of a better word, is pushed up to the heart, this is the point that it all gets a bit science fiction and rather scary, terribly intimidating as people mill around you doing their thing but not really explaining much to you.

A contrast liquid is used, no, I didn't ask what it was, but when your chest is viewed through a scanner / x ray style machine, the definition is incredibly accurate and I laid there watching this procedure in real time, I think I could actually feel the wire touch my heart, the heart has nerve ends and can feel, most of your insides cannot.

This procedure dispelled an age old myth, my last wife had called me heartless, it was now proven, I did in fact have one.

I was, 1 hour later, being wheeled in a bed back to the ward with a heavy sand bag laid against the wound area to apply extra pressure until the bleeding had stopped and told that I had to lie still and flat for the next four hours, the staff gradually raise the back of the bed during the day until you are fully sat up, they also seem to take it in turns to look at your bollocks every hour to see if you are bleeding, quite embarrassing when they have a shift change and someone you haven't met walks up, whips back the blanket, takes a peek at your bollocks and walks off..

I had to patiently wait for my results which didn't arrive, instead a nasty bout of stomach disorders swept throughout the wards and no one was allowed in or out until they had identified the problem and dealt with it.

This meant I was left to sit in this infected ward with a bunch of strangers until such time as the infection was deemed safe, no one could tell me what was going on, so I got dressed and went home as at this time I was not aware of how ill I was and I was keen to get back to work.

I had not yet developed any patience or tolerance, manners or well being towards the hospital staff that were doing their very best for me, if only I could see it into the future I would have behaved very differently.

The following day I was feeling well enough for work so I went round a couple of sites and then had an appointment with my bank manager.

I was just going into the bank when my mobile phone rang and the gentleman who had carried out my Angio gram was discussing with me what was going on, he was young, charming, Mr Andrew Money-Koyle and I was to have a few conversations with him and meet up again a year down the road.

He asked me where I was and what I was doing; he seemed terribly concerned and apologised for not getting to see me while I was still on the ward at the hospital, some cock up or other had prevented his visit.

He said, having reviewed my report, that nothing could be done for me in his field, ie, Angio Plasti was out of the question and I was in need of a quadruple heart by pass which obviously meant open heart surgery and he advised me to go home, stop driving and the hospital would be in touch very soon as it was his opinion that I was now very much at risk of a heart attack or stroke, my arteries all showing blockages and narrowing restricting the flow of blood to my heart muscle. Ooh that sounds nasty.

I have to admit this all came as quite a shock, even after waiting for nearly forty years for this news, it still came as a huge shock to me that it was finally about to happen, I had succumbed to the family curse and I was bloody scared.

I didn't have to wait very long to get into hospital, I had no sooner got home and had a chat with Linda, had my tea and settled down for the evening when it all started off again, this time massive chest pain, big fat lady sitting on my chest, buzzing in my ears and the usual aches down my arms and face, I decided against having my evening cigarette and decided to lie down and die instead, Linda wouldn't let me though.

It is very frightening when you cannot get your breath, when you cannot breathe in because of the amount of weight on your chest, when you are passing into unconsciousness and losing control.

Linda called the ambulance, yes we did get the fire brigade instead, and this time, being a heart case, I was taken to the John Radcliffe NHS trust hospital in Oxford which was to become my home for the next two months, Linda following on in her car as always, the ambulance playing its merry little tune and flashing blue lights all the way, me in the back chucking my guts up and thinking I was definitely dying this time and I must admit, not a little scared, I was now very scared, no more bravado, no more devil may care, I have run out of funny things to say, this was me, this is happening right here, right now to me, oh my God, did I want my mum.

Chapter four

The John Radcliffe NHS Trust (JR) which is situated on top of a hill on the North East side of Oxford city, is a huge great sprawling mass of conflicting structures, randomly thrown together, started in the 1970,s I believe, and continuing to develop even to this day, it was to my loss that I was too early to get to stay in the brand new centre of excellence heart centre, I had to put up with the far less special centre of no particular qualification, old and quite grubby, in the basement of the existing seven story building, made the more confusing because the entrance is on level two, the A&E department being on level one with the cardiac services below that.

It is a huge hospital, with the usual small and very expensive car parks, difficult access and almost no facilities but hey ho, this time I really did need to be there, this time it was for real, I was facing the man who dresses in a black robe and carries a scythe around, I didn't have a pot to call my own and wasn't sure if I could pay the ferry man should this all go tits up.

I was very aware of my mortality, I was alone, the way that I had come into the world, alone and rather concerned for tomorrow.

Linda was very soon sitting along side me and there was plenty of staff but I still was feeling very alone, where I was looking at going I would be going on my own and no amount of "you will be all right" was going to lift my mood, not today anyway, I was feeling somewhat sorry for myself at this point.

I was deposited by the wonderful ambulance staff in the A&E department where I was immediately set upon, I expect much to the annoyance of the multitude of people waiting to be seen, it is not that my case was more important, only that it was obviously more urgent and in all hospitals need is the key to timing, if you have a spot on your arse, this is not the place to come to get it seen to and the A&E staff take a very dim view on dealing with minor injuries and irritations, in more than one sense. If I had been drunk or fighting or both, I do believe I would prefer to keep it to myself rather than suffer the verbal scalding handed out in A&E

I received the usual top up of morphine, fluids, ECG and blood tests for starters and was nodding off, pain free and by some miracle, anxiety free now that I was in the right place, safe, it is just like going to the dentist, the moment that you get to the hospital, the pain stops.

They called High Wycombe and managed to get the report on my very recent scans and I was given a lot of drugs, injections and blood thinning tablets which are designed to help avoid the possible follow up stroke and left to sleep for a while so that they could get my bloods checked to see if a marker was present which would indicate a recent heart event, there was not.

Linda, bless her, always by my side, wouldn't go home even though it was by now past midnight and I was beginning to worry about her, she was scared, like me, and she was very tired. I do not like her driving at night, she is a timid driver and I would worry till she was safely home.

I managed to get her to see sense, the staff told her that I would still be around in the morning and that she needed to look after her self so she went off home, I managed to get a text off to her to say good night and she seemed OK, or as ok as one can be when the shit hits the fan.

The blood tests are repeated quite frequently because an enzyme is found in your blood if you have had a major trauma like a heart attack and they keep taking blood for eight hours, sometimes twelve.

I was put into Cardiac services unit which I believe is on the 1st floor, could be the second as it is such a confusing place and given another going over by doctors and nurses even though it was well past bed time, I was fed and watered, sandwiches and tea, then dressed in a gown, undressed more like as they are far to small and always leave my arse hanging out, at least I was allowed to trot to the bathroom alone, providing I promised to conceal my rather spotty arse that is.

I took to wearing this one size fits all gown backwards with a second gown the right way round so that I was covered from all angles, didn't want to upset anyone in the new mixed ward scheme, old lady dies as half naked man staggers by the end of her bed.

They gave me a telemetry devise to wear, it hung from a cord around the neck, which, coupled with the stick on ECG tabs, a blood pressure wrap round my upper right arm and a blood oxygen meter on my left hand little finger, could monitor my heart, pulse and oxygen throughout the day and night and transmitted the data to a computer which the doctors and more importantly, the consultants and surgeons could look at and diagnose my condition more thoroughly, I stayed here for three days and nights while they stabilised my condition and recorded the data required.

It is so difficult to do everything half sat up, not allowed to lie flat because of fluid build up on the lungs and not allowed to sit up because of all the equipment that you are wearing, at all times attached to a metering device for drugs and this was also the first time that I had been put onto insulin, I was no longer self administering my drugs, they were doing it all now, more often by machine, remotely.

I also had to have an injection into my belly everyday, it hurt or rather stung very badly and left a huge black / blue bruise each and every time that it was administered, this I came to hate but nearly all of us on the ward had to have it because it was a blood conditioner, anti clot stuff and was very much par for the course and it was universally detested by all.

The nurses would check my blood sugar levels every three or four hours, even through the night while I slept but they always managed to shove the needle in so far that I would bleed for ages, when I do it with my own machine I seldom even need to wipe my finger afterwards.

Then the bad times started, I was moved up to the long stay wards on the seventh floor, purgatory in concrete.

I was disgusted as soon as the lift doors opened, the smell, the filth and total lack of care which seemed to be the over riding factor about the place, it looked a hundred years old and stank to high heaven of human beings, vomit, shit and urine with noise pollution being the biggest factor of all.

People were pressing their call buttons and calling out, being ignored and calling again and again, my very first impressions of this place made my heart slump, my spirits just fell away and I could have cried like a baby.

The wards are made up of six beds per unit with about sixteen or more units per floor and both the sixth floor and the seventh floor were used for general medicine and long stay patients several hundred at a time.

The JR is also a teaching hospital with a huge amount of staff who attends the wards for at least twelve hours a day, ten people visit you and almost all will be student doctors.

While I appreciated that I was in an NHS hospital, I had previously always had private health care, I was over whelmed by the lack of care, the amount of elderly people who should really have been at home looked after by their families but given the state of the nation, the elderly end up staying in the hospital because of their children not wanting to help them or having to go to work to keep their own children, and a complete lack of home services and this obviously was not taken into account with the amount of staff on duty at any one time, they just couldn't cope, far to much going on for half a dozen or so nurses per floor with this many aged and immobile people.

I am not being rude to the people who leave their parents in here, they probably do not have a choice and have to go to work, I blame the system for not making it possible for children to look after their own due to funding issues, there should be a generous carers allowance, it would avoid all of this heart break for old people who I doubt would want to be in this hell hole, most of the inmates, I am told, could be looked after at home, if their children could afford the time to do so and the system provided enough nursing care in the community.

Food was being served now, I think it was food, it didn't either look good nor taste good and I waited for my beloved to find me and get me something better, I am sorry to say that I have always eaten very well, Linda is a good cook as am I.

What really stuck in my throat was that food was put down in front of old people who couldn't or wouldn't feed them selves and there was never enough staff or helpers to feed them so a lot of people had cold food at every meal and some had no food at all and while I could choose not to eat this muck, to some people this was all that they were likely to get so it not only became important if they were to keep their strength up it also became the high light of the day for them.

Now let's get onto the nutters, the loonies and those that are unaware that they are supposed to be dead.

While I understand the reasoning that nutters become ill and have to, on occasion, be admitted to hospital, I do find it really hard to believe that they all seem to gravitate towards me, it cannot be an accident.

It cannot be possible that every time I go to the hospital, sit on a bus or stand in a queue I always collect a nutter, they seem to believe that I actually want to communicate with them, that I give a toss.

Why, when I am obviously intolerant, am I subjected to this form of torture, why are they right next to or more often than not in the bed in front of me where I can see them, they can see me and start smiling and calling out to me, like I care.

I am not aware that I may have a friendly face, and that somehow I communicate to them that I too am lonely, that I will listen to their problems, that I will not kill them in their sleep and eat them.

This time of going into hospital was no different, I got a nutter, it wasn't his fault because, bless him, he got me.

His name was John, they all seem to be called John, he couldn't see but instead of quietly lying in bed not being able to see, he called out every two minutes "nurse, nurse, I cant see " at the top of his voice.

What no one had explained to him, not in the last minute or so which seemed to be the length of his attention span and memory, was that he wasn't supposed to see, he was blind, and had been for the past ten years yet he deemed it necessary to call out day and night, even when it was too dark to see, that he could not see and no amount of telling him was going to change his mind about it, he had made up his mind not to see sense.

He had more attention than the rest of the ward put together in an effort to stop me from getting out of my bed and killing him in his sleep, on the very rare occasion that he did sleep, and in the end the staff moved me along the corridor to a quiet little unit with a lot of very content and quiet other chaps, though it was still possible to hear John calling for sight, but like his dinner, he didn't get any.

However, during the night the porters moved one quiet little old man out of my recently found haven, just because he had died, he wasn't making a fuss so why couldn't they just leave him alone, I hadn't even had the time to exchange pleasantries with him, and they replaced him with another nutter.

This one was something else, barking mad and refused to stay in his bed, wouldn't stop wandering around even though quite clearly he wasn't fit to be walking about unassisted, clearly had mad cows disease or something.

He must have tipped the scales at something over thirty stones, was in excess of six feet six inches tall, and round, and must have been in his late fifties.

It was plain to see that he had heart issues due to the blackness and swelling of his legs which looked like a pair of very bruised scrotums, all wrinkled and black.

He had the most unpleasant of habits in that he would wander around while shitting himself, it running down his legs and onto the floor, if the staff could keep him in bed, he would have to be changed on the hour and he made the place stink to high heaven, he had no idea that he was doing it, it was like watching a cow walking around in a field, thank God he didn't have a tail or it would have flicked everywhere.

He came over to my bed and with a toothless grin offered me his hand as a hello, his hand was covered in shit which he proceeded to wipe down my curtains, I am sure that you can imagine my response, I went berserk pressing every button I could find and removed all of my sensors in an attempt to get out of bed and away from him as he was so keen to touch me.

The nurses came running and removed him, I was having an absolute fit, my monitors were going through the roof and there in front of me was this grinning pile of shit who appeared to have the mental ability of an old dining chair.

After everything had calmed down the staff nurses, with the help of some porters, moved this chap out of the ward, my protestations were very valid, as far as I was concerned the duty of care had been misplaced and I was making so much fuss it would put peoples names off of the Christmas card list for good, I wanted an enquiry and wanted the united nations and NATO involved, I was so bloody angry, I felt violated and abused, contaminated and at risk, he scared the living shit out of me.

Now don't get me wrong here, I am a very large man myself and have been trained in the art of hurting people but it is an unwritten rule that one does not spank the loonies of this world and what makes it all so frightening is that you have to back away all of the time because if you do lose it with a loony or someone smaller than yourself, someone who cannot defend them selves, you are the baddy.

Mr barking mad was moved to a side room where he spent the night on the floor beside his bed covered in his own shit and urine, this was his choice and the busy staff appeared to leave him to get on with it because he was so big and strong that he had to be attended to mob handed and there just wasn't enough staff on duty to deal with him.

The cleaning staff had to go through the whole ward, again, including the removal of my curtains, I made them wash everything down and make the smell go away, peace and quiet at last, we thought for I was not alone in my protestations, the whole ward had had enough and he had only been here a few hours and I had seemingly been elected a spokes person, a voice for the other poor buggers that would normally have put up with this intolerable situation.

But no, when fatty shit bag saw the young lady up a step ladder hanging a clean set of curtains around my bed it was just to much for him, he was out of the side room and raced over to where the young Polish girl was up the step ladder, I say raced, I have seen thorn bushed move faster, and grabbing the ladder he tipped her onto the end of my bed, I don't speak Polish but the air was blue, she set my heart racing, the bells went off, he was removed and the following day there was an enquiry.

Looking back on this incident I find myself struggling to keep a straight face, it is something out of a "carry on" film, it is just too outrageous.

I am adamant that this behaviour with nutters, loonies and people who point blank refuse to die, is not conducive towards my well being in this place where I now find myself trapped and that the NHS is doing me an injustice and bad practices exist taking advantage of my vulnerability. I am stuck in bed while loonies and the undead walk free around me, looking at me, talking to me, it is not unreasonable to feel slightly put upon.

I have worked in the Central Middlesex Hospital, West London where loons etc have their own wing and staffing levels and procedures and geared up to cater for the problems, they do not mix loons and normal people so do not have conflict, the JR would do well to look at other institutional policies as my care has been seriously effected by this stress and extreme unhappiness which should have been avoided, and yes I do fully understand the principles of financial constraints as much as I understand management cock ups.

Generally the nursing staff have proven to be very kind and go about their business as quietly and efficiently as is possible given the shortage of staff.

They are very mixed in race, there does seem to be someone from every continent if not country in the world, Chinese, Philippine, Malayan, Polish, German, Welsh as well as the normal Indian and Caribbean contingents and a language barrier most definitely exists as does the mixed and varied levels of training and general attitudes.

There is also a full contingent of male nurses, some gay some not and some not at all sure as well as quite a few ginger people, but enough said about them.

The Asians always seem to be the most gentle and smile far more than their European counterparts and do not seem to get into a sweat, a laid back attitude seems to prevail and it is very difficult to tell any ones rank as the uniforms seem to be wear what you like, some wear theatre kit, others wear whites, sisters generally are in dark blue with some staff nurses in blue, green or white.

The cleaning staff are all Eastern European, very few speaking any English and if you can speak some English you get promoted to dishing out tea and breakfast in the mornings, it is not though, always obvious who you are talking to and on more than one occasion I asked for a pee bottle and got a cup of tea.

The days march on, the food is crap, the loonies will not die and I feel time has come to do something about this very unpleasant place that I find myself in, I am drained both physically and mentally, I am not at all used to being unhappy and find I cannot do anything about it.

I have decided to get out of here, I think I have been here for two weeks now and clearly as I will not survive if I leave the hospital I must at the very least take back some control and a plan is hatched, a very cunning plan.

I get out of my bed before breakfast comes round, put on my fluffy grey dressing gown over bed shorts and tee shirt and put on my slippers, I am off for a huge adventure and I am not at all sure where it will take me, not even sure if I will get there alive.

I walk across to the fire doors and through to the stairs, metal steps covered with a dirty grey vinyl with painted metal balustrade and plastic coated hand rail, it will bloody well hurt if I do fall over, anyway down I go, three floors and about turn, making sure that I am alone, up I go as fast as my weak carcass can carry me to arrive at the seventh floor puffing and panting and fat ladies dancing on my chest, I am sprawled on the ward floor with all hell breaking loose around me, I am conscious, I am unconscious, I can see, now I cannot see, the buzzing in my head is so loud that I cannot hear what is being said, round one to me, I have survived the trip and now they are getting me into bed and an oxygen mask is going on, ECG stickers and all wired up again, a needle is going in, more morphine and soon off to sleep, dreaming of the dirty once white walls and damp stained ceilings of the staircase.

I wake to find my curtains are still closed around my bed, I am being told off, scolded by the staff nurse but I don't care, it was an adventure, an outing, I went on holiday for a few minutes and I made it back.

The staff nurse had said "you gave me such a fright" I said " gave you such a fright, how do you think I was feeling"

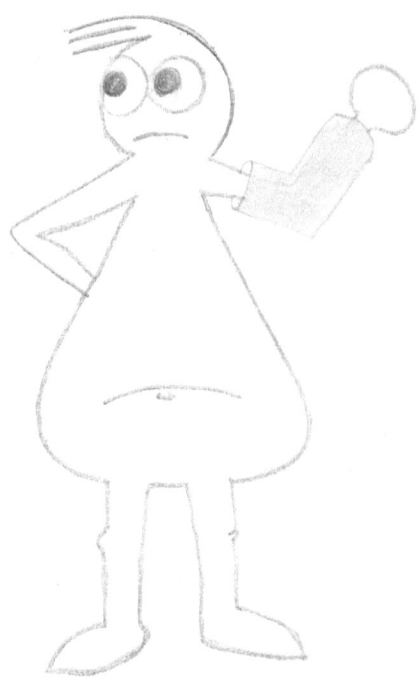

Chapter five

The next day, straight after breakfast and tablets I start another chapter of my journey, down to cardiac services, the heart ward where I am to stay until my operation, my prank, as dangerous as it was, brought me up the list and although that is selfish, it was one hell of a risk to take so I am chuffed that it worked out for me, chuffed that I have got away from the nutters but now not so chuffed that I have brought my Armageddon closer.

I am asked a couple of times by the nurse why I keep smiling, but I cannot tell them it is because they don't give loonies heart surgery, there are not any here and all is peaceful and quiet, orderly and professional.

I think the staff get you all wound up in a noisy, smelly ward on purpose so that when your turn does come round you actually look forward to going into theatre, anything to get away from the wards, facing my nemesis was a doddle compared to being upstairs and facing those bloody lunatics day in day out.

I only had one single waiting day on the heart ward, just one day to explore and acclimatise to my new surroundings, see the sights and meet the people

It was deathly quiet all of the time with enforced rest periods when everyone was encouraged to sleep, to rest, no one was shouting or calling out.

There was staff everywhere, the ratio during the day seemed something like one nurse for every three or four patients, very different from upstairs where the ratio was more like one nurse for every twenty patients and that is not counting the very high volume of doctors, anaesthetists, physiotherapists, clinical care operatives and general dogs bodies.

I was still connected to the insulin machinery and other drugs were being regularly pumped into me in preparation for the operation, the machine being attached to a wheeled trolley, like a stand and it had to go everywhere with me so I never felt lonely, I even thought of giving it a name.

The ward was old fashioned in décor with a mix of pre finished plastic panels and polished hard wood dado with dark non slip vinyl flooring and pastel emulsion finishes elsewhere, white ceiling tiles, strip lights and awful flowery curtains around the beds all feeling like it had been designed by Stevie Wonder on crack cocaine.

The equipment as quite good, all the beds were electric and had multiple adjustment which made for a good deal of comfort, there was a tea or coffee point, a visitors room as well as a nice relaxation area which was surprisingly well stocked with books and magazines.

The bathrooms were particularly terrible with bright pink tiles from floor to ceiling offset by dark grey non slip vinyl flooring and bad cheap and nasty lighting.

These details were to prove important to me in the future, very important indeed and I am glad that I had plenty of time to take it all in.

In the cubicle that I was later to occupy following my surgery, was a chap late twenties, average build, who had under gone heart surgery and he was sitting in the plastic / vinyl covered easy chair next to his bed and as I walked past him on my way to the bathroom our eyes met so I stopped to pass the time.

It never ceases to amaze me how, when in adversity, men tend towards each other, gather together in a common cause, no matter what that cause, safety in numbers even when it is surgery which is neither a team sport nor audience participation, we still like to have others near who have shared our problem.

He had quite a few pipes sticking out of him draining into bottles beside the bed, a wire or two but nothing as bad as I had been led to believe, he looked like a bit actor from Star trek, a Borg.

When I asked him how long ago he had been to theatre I was staggered by his reply, he had been for heart surgery the day before, had a valve replacement and here he was sat up in the chair reading his news paper, I was gob smacked, I had been expecting him to say four of five days, I wouldn't have been surprised had he said a week but no, one single day.

I was elated when Linda came to visit and told her of my conversation and my expectations for the same, I was not to know what was to come nor how long before I was to be able to sit in a chair and hold a news paper.

In the bed next to me was a chap called Dave Wise, a lovely man who's claim to fame was that he was the proud owner of the oldest pace maker in existence that was still working inside some ones body and he had come in to get it replaced after nearly twenty years of good service, I joked with him that it must have been made in Japan because had it been made in the UK it would have gone on strike after a couple of weeks.

He also had a swelling of the Aorta, the area above the heart, that he was hoping they could also sort out at the same time but sadly Dave had to wait for nearly three months in hospital before he was deemed well enough to undergo his surgery, which he thankfully survived.

Dave's wife didn't drive and had restricted access, relying on relatives to bring her the twenty miles from where they lived in Reading, Berkshire, all the way to the hospital, so Dave had to rely on what the ward dished up for his meals and treats were very rare.

Linda was always very keen to supply me with a varied and interesting diet and my being in hospital was no reason for this to change so she would cart in all sorts of goodies, my favourite being bagels with smoked salmon and cream cheese filling which I did not share with anyone, they were my treat.

She would knock up salads and dressings, cold meats and pies and always brought me small sachets of salt and pepper.

These condiments could transform the very bland meals served up by the hospital and word got round that I had salt, a banned substance on a cardiac ward, and I became very popular with visitors to my bed and goodies exchanged for said salt, I was to become known as the white powder man and made many a friend because of this basic but needed product.

Linda, recognising Dave's plight, brought him in a cold beef salad so that he could refuse the awful stuff supplied and he got stuck in with gusto only to have his wife turn up unexpectedly with both of their adult children and four grandchildren who all sat down and watched him devour his meal, he couldn't stop because Linda wanted to take the plates home.

Dave was to become a firm friend in the future and I visit him on occasion, not often enough though.

He caught a bit of skin cancer on the top of his head recently which the local hospital has been unable to treat, the skin graft fell off and he has to wear a hat all of the time, even in bed.

Being a nice bloke, I have promised him my hairy scrotum to patch his head up if I die first.

That evening Linda and I spent a few quiet moments with my cubicle curtains drawn, we needed to say good bye as she wouldn't be along again until after I had been for surgery.

We had only been together a few months, March to December, we hardly knew each other in the bigger scheme of things and this was a really big ask, it really was an immense undertaking on Linda's part to sit through this.

We tried to laugh it off and make big plans for when I came home but as my father had died during heart surgery I knew that she was aware that I was rather nervous and didn't expect to be coming home again, I couldn't make too much small talk which must have been refreshing for her because it is normally so hard to shut me up.

We held each other quietly for a while.

She left rather late to go home, I almost had to chase her out of the ward and I settled down with my book, steam engines or something rather neutral.

I had a late evening visit from the anaesthetist who talked me through a few things but I really wasn't listening, he gave me a sleeping tablet and left me to my thoughts, which I wasn't too keen on, I was having nightmares and I hadn't even got off to sleep yet.

Surprisingly I had a really good nights sleep and was woken at six am next morning to prepare for surgery, a very thorough shower using a bright red surgical sterile liquid body wash and then some pre med needles in my bottom, I could have killed a cup of tea but was not allowed food nor drink.

I got myself dressed in the usual paper hat, paper pants and a gown that was far too small and was covered in flowers, how very gay.

The consultant surgeon and consultant anaesthetist paid a visit and talked me through the paperwork which I signed without reading, they tried to discuss the risks but I didn't want to know, they tried to discuss the surgery and equally I really didn't want to know about that either.

I had decided that there was absolutely nothing that I could say or do that would change what they had to do to me or that would change my risk so it was best to let them just get on with it, I was at this time completely full of faith in their ability to do the best they could, with what they had, ie me, they could only do so much then so I signed on the dotted line, signed for them to do what ever they deemed necessary to make me well or at the very least keep me alive.

I was moved sideways from my bed onto a trolley feeling rather conscious about the paper hat and pants that I was displaying and quietly wheeled down to the theatre, I am sure we used a lift but am not aware of going up nor down as before, I was quite lost and arrived at the theatre feeling as high as a kite and best part asleep, warm and rather cosy.

I lay on the trolley thinking two things, the first being, given my enormous bulk, how are they going to move me from this trolley onto an operating table when I am asleep and cannot help and the second thing was how much it would take or cost to paint all the chips in the walls and doors caused by the edges of the trolleys, off white always looks so dirty…they needed nice soft pastel shades.

Needles were stuck into my hands and taped into place and the staff moved up a gear and after a few questions and answers to again confirm my identity, I had to confirm my signature on the consent forms, I was sent to the land of nod, for a very, very long time.

Chapter six

I am being watched, I think I am awake.
I feel nothing; can see nothing, falling into darkness

I was being watched, someone was touching me, I am trying to move but cannot, I see a ceiling with lights on, a voice says "lie still Andrew".
Who is this Andrew they are talking to.

I am trying to move but cannot, something touches me and I am falling again, falling into sleep, someone is speaking to me but they seem such a long way away now.

I awake and feel that something or someone is touching me, watching me, I can see lights, a ceiling, it is going black again, and I am falling, frightened.
I am told to keep still.

This goes on for seven nights and seven days, I couldn't count them at the time for each time I woke I didn't remember the last, I was terrified, I had no idea where I was, who I was or what I was though I was aware that I could neither move nor speak, was I dead, is this dead, I don't remember hearing a fat lady sing.

I was awake, awake but not awake…

I still couldn't move, couldn't see, couldn't speak.

I heard something near me and tried to call out, no sound came out, someone told me to lie still.

I found that I could only move my right leg, I could only partly feel my right leg below the knee and it was sore, but soon my sight was beginning to return, blurred and closed in, no peripheral vision to speak of, if I could speak that is, I still couldn't.

I lifted my leg up and down banging it on the bed and a nurse came into view and told me to lie still, well that answered a question, I am in a hospital, or someone likes dressing up. It also asked more questions, why am I in hospital, where is this hospital. Who am I.

I couldn't speak properly but could make out one wheezing word per lung full of air and asked where, who and what and she told me that I have had an operation and again to lie still for a while, no I mustn't lie down I had to stay semi sat up.

My sight was by now returning and I could see my body stretched out in front of me and my God what a bloody mess, what the hell had happened to me.

I was cut from my throat down to my stomach which was all stitched up with three huge pipes coming from my abdomen and draining beneath me somewhere into something I assumed.

I had an even bigger pipe coming out of my cock and going in the same direction as the others and I can remember thinking that I am grateful that I was not awake while that was pushed up there, it was huge, like a garden hose and corrugated, held to my cock with what I assumed to be sticky tape.

I had a drain pipe from my groin where I had a huge wound , a pipe from my neck, wires sticking out of my neck and pipes going into both arms, water, food, anti-biotic and insulin, I was later told.

I was cut from my right ankle up to the knee and this had about twenty rather large stitches, and from my left foot right up to my groin again all stitched up with far more stitches than I was able to count.

I was very sore around my bottom area, between my bum cheeks, bed sores and again really red raw behind my neck where quite a chunk of skin had been rubbed off, where they have secured the breathing kit to my head.

I was still completely unaware what had happened to me but found it so difficult to speak that I just couldn't get the question across even had the nurse had the time or interest in listening to me and I just dozed for an hour or two, waiting until the time was right.

The nurse was reminding me to sit up again, gravity was in control, not me, I couldn't sit up if I wanted to, I really wanted to lie down and sleep had I been given the option.

The nurse came to me and fitted a mask around my face, removing the oxygen mask that I was quite happily using at the time, she still didn't bother to speak to me other than to tell me to be quiet and keep still.

This new mask had an attachment on the side which when installed with a cartridge acted as an inhaler, it was absolutely bloody awful, it was like breathing powder and I found the whole mask completely claustrophobic and struggled to complete each of the cartridges, struggling with uncontrollable arms to yank the mask off with the nurses trying to make me keep it on, telling me that I really had to have the medicine that it contained.

Although I eventually had to have the medicine it was something that I really struggled with, the rubber smell of the mask reminding me of the dentist when I was quite young.

I was feeling terrible, I had woken in pain and fear for I knew nothing of where I was nor what had happened to me, I was incredibly nauseous, I wanted to be sick but couldn't hold onto the sick bowl, my hands didn't belong to me any more, I was dizzy and wanted to just go back to sleep but they wouldn't let me, I had to stay awake, I was not going to be allowed to lie down again and was scolded every time that I slid down the bed, I couldn't prevent it as I couldn't feel my legs yet.

I could hear the nurse talking to her friend on the telephone complaining bitterly that there had been a mess up with her pay cheque and she was furious, I know she was furious, she was taking it out on me, the unfriendly bitch.

I was sat there trying to think but couldn't think, I couldn't think of anything to think about, my memory banks were completely asleep and I was just in a fog, lost in a fog of nothing to think about, it was incredible, not able to think about anything, not able to remember anything, knowing nothing.

I was glancing around and saw someone I thought I recognised," I know you," I struggled to say, no one could hear me anyway but it was my Linda and she was coming over to me, I just burst into tears, I still had no idea what was going on, why was I so confused, why couldn't I speak or move about, why couldn't I think.

She carefully explained to me that I had undergone a quadruple heart by-pass and they had elected to keep me asleep because they felt that I had a chest infection and preferred to restrict my movements and that I hadn't moved for seven days and nights, this was day eight post operation.

This explained to me what I thought had been dreams were in fact real, I had been lying here all of this time, I had been spoken to night after night when they had checked me over before sending me back off to sleep, all the time thinking that I had been abducted by aliens or worse, Ginger Welsh people and they would teach me never to use a vowel again.

Finally I had the answers, Linda explained it all to me, I had partial memory failure, I couldn't think straight and it was all because of the anaesthetic that they had been using on me for more than a week now and it also explained why none of my limbs would respond to my instructions to move, they were still fast asleep and hopefully normality will return given time, normal service will resume.

It was quite astonishing how Linda turning up has changed things, apart from now knowing what the hell was going on, I didn't feel as though I was alone anymore, I knew that she wouldn't let them do anything to me that they shouldn't.

It is amazing how pathetic I have become, I cannot move, cannot speak very well, cannot even sit up in bed and have to be protected and monitored all of the time.

How can they do this to someone and yet they survive, can my body ever get over all of these dreadful injuries, will I ever walk out of this place?

The anaesthetist paid me a visit and gave me some tablets to swallow which I just could not get down, I couldn't even manage the water without violent coughing bouts, something that is not recommended following open heart surgery, it bloody hurts.

He took a look down my throat and could see that the flap across my lung / stomach pipes was damaged and I couldn't swallow without something going into my lungs, oh dear. This had been caused by the oxygen pipe that had been stuck down my throat for more than a week now, I suppose one is not supposed to have something stuck down your throat for more than a week.

He advised the importance of my taking the tablets and insisted that I must also have food and trotted off to get some feeding pipes with every intention of stuffing them up my nose and down into my stomach so that I could be liquid fed.

I did ask if he would mind leaving me alone until I was feeling a bit better but he had the scent now and was not to be deterred from his new project.

With Linda holding onto me he presented this pipe to my left nostril and started to push it in, it wasn't going to happen and he pushed some more insinuating that I wasn't trying even though I could feel the tears rolling down my face, no I wasn't crying, I couldn't really feel anything being still quite numb, it wasn't as though there was anything that I could either do to help or hinder the pipe going in, it just wouldn't and he was getting more and more upset by my apparent refusal to let him shove pipes up my nose.

He popped off again and came back with a syringe full of anaesthetic which he promptly started to inject into my nose, as if I wasn't already half dead, and started pushing again, very much against my will I might add and once I had a nose bleed he started to shove it into my right nostril which pissed me off even further, my nose was now full of anaesthetic gel and blood which I couldn't breath through and I was now very annoyed and Linda was getting upset because of my obvious distress.

I had had enough and told him, rather wheezed at him to sod off and leave me in peace, now he was pissed off.

He told me that if he couldn't get the food into my stomach, I would not be able to take the tablets, he insisted that he had to get the pipes into my nose but I had already had far more than I could take and he was forced to back down, though to my dismay he was visibly angry about it, took it all very personally, oh dear.

I asked him, as a closing shot, how I had been taking my drugs while I had been in my enforced coma during the past week, without a response from him, arrogant bastard, I hadn't exactly been chewing them up had I, maybe that explains my rather sore arse...

I was destined to remain hungry and thirsty for the immediate future as I just could not swallow anything without violent and prolonged coughing which given that my chest was only held together by a few twists of silver wire and a few stitches really was not a great idea.

Linda and I chatted softly, she was visibly tired but also elated that I had woken up at last and she could feel that I would now survive the procedure

I had not been aware that she had been sitting next to my bed for many hours each day, talking to me, loving me and wishing me well, I had not known, had not heard her and not felt her gently caressing me, helping me through this most desperate of times, not knowing if I would wake up or worse wake up a vegetable. I was also completely unaware that she had no knowledge that I wore false teeth, she knew now as I had six top teeth on a metal plate and they were all missing...oops.

Before she went off home for the night we were paid a visit by one of the cardiac team, Professor Taggarts main man, who had assisted as they performed the surgery and all was ok, good news all round because the quadruple by-pass had gone well and a full recovery was expected, though due to the size of my chest and arms concern had been expressed as to my recovery time.

I did find it rather annoying the way I was introduced, the consultant would point at me and say "Andrew Kingston, cabbage" and then go off into lots of technical jargon and it was a few days before I asked the question, "why do they keep calling me a cabbage".

It was eventually explained to me by the staff nurse, staff nurses do everything on the cardiac wards, in fact I doubt if you get on this ward without being at least that grade, she explained to me that they were not being rude, CaBaGe spelt out Cardiac Artery Bypass Grafts and then they would normally add the number of grafts done, ie double, triple or in my case quadruple.

Obviously the more grafts done the harder the job, the longer on the operating table and the more mobile the heart would have to be, they actually pull it out and virtually rest it on your shoulder, repair it and stuff it all back in again, reminds me of my days at the slaughter house except we didn't wait for them to wake up again. I was feeling as though they had played couple of sides of volley ball with mine before shoving it back in.

Linda, bless her, went of home and I went off to sleep, hungry, thirsty, confused but alive.

During the night I was well awake, I had slept for so long over the past week that I suppose I didn't really need anymore.

It is quite amazing how you can find an additional dozen hours or more when you cannot sleep; the night seems to go on and on and on

I entertained myself by trying to day dream, but all dreams are based on accumulated information and as I had information melt down I just lay there trying to think, I couldn't manage it.

I did however feel in need of the lavatory, my urine was nicely being cared for by my beautiful little piss pipe but I could really do with emptying the other end and according to the rules of engagement summoned a nurse.

The lady that turned up proved to be more than just a nurse, she was an absolute angel to me throughout the whole night, taking far more time and care than the day staff had bothered with, maybe her pay cheque was correct.

She kindly and gently reminded me that because I had eaten nothing for more than a week it would, in her experience, be highly unlikely that I have any solids in me, ie I am without stools and laughing she trotted off.

I gave it a while until I was sure and called her again, I had a call button fixed to my hand with tape so that I could neither lose it nor drop it , she attended again and reminded me of our previous conversations.

I insisted that I think I am getting uncomfortable, I think because to be honest I wasn't sure if or what I could actually feel at this stage and it could have just been the sensation of feeling coming back but she once again assured me that I only had wind, quite normal given the amount of drugs used on me lately she agreed, I on the other hand didn't share her confidence.

I persisted with my insistence and along with two other nurses, both male heterosexual and German, I was hoisted onto a very cold and very uncomfortable metal bed pan into which I did the noisiest fart I have ever heard, echoed around the metal bed pan and all around the ward like a huge church organ, her point taken and I was ceremonially removed from said bed pan never to request one again as the experience is both painful and very embarrassing.

I gave it half an hour and the above was repeated again, just wind and I dropped off to sleep feeling outdone and the lady nurse rather pleased with herself for being in the know.

It is astonishingly difficult to be man handled especially when you are on the wrong side of twenty stone, the human body does not come with handles, love handles excluded here, and there is only so much that you can get hold of when trying to lift someone. Factor into that equation the severity of the wounds and you will see that they are not too keen on moving you about.

Apparently, I could piss for England, as soon as they put up another bag of liquid drip, it would have gone right through me into my drain bottle, it was quite unusually fast the amount of liquid I used, in my prime, I could drink three pints of beer without needing the toilet, now I need the toilet if I think about beer.

I woke later in the night, all was quiet and peaceful, I was sure I needed the toilet but given the earlier lessons decided that it would be far less painful if I were to sneak out a crafty fart in peace, it was excruciatingly painful being manhandled on and off of a bed pan because I couldn't help and due to my weight, nearly dead weight at that I was hoisted up and down quite violently with a one, two three, go, owe.

My sneaky little fart turned into a nightmare as I shit everywhere, it was like new born baby poo, no solids just poo and it went up my back as well as down my legs, all over my wounds and onto the floor.

I pressed my button and the staff turned up, laughing quite openly even though they had agreed it couldn't happen, not a bit of annoyance with the amount of mess. One must consider how long that mess had been brewing inside me to be able to envisage the full effect.

I had to be rolled onto my side while I was washed and the bed sheets changed, first one side and then the other, I couldn't breath while I was on my side and was in terrible pain, my oxygen censor being the controlling factor, when it set off the alarms they would let me back onto my back to breath for a short while.

The funniest thing about this uncomfortable time was the Germans taking the Mickey, apparently the lady nurse was a Lesbian so they insisted that she should get the practice in by washing my cock, and then the two German lads started on me with " you may have won zee war but you are not in control now are you" all sorted out with as much fun as possible, a really good bunch of people, just what the doctor ordered, excuse the pun.

The nurse, Sue, hung around and chatted with me to make sure I was alright and that my signs all returned to normal and we talked about what had happened earlier with the rather unfriendly anaesthetist.

She volunteered the chance that they may have some cartons of milk shake and would fetch some for me if I would like to give it a go, I was well up for that and off she trotted.

She brought two 300ml cartons of long life Strawberry milk shake and some drinking straws, I only knew the flavour of the milk because she told me, I could tastes absolutely nothing and usually I cannot bear the taste of UHT milk products so it was a blessing that I could taste nothing.

The only way that I could manage to drink any was by sitting up and forward as much as possible and getting a little of the milk onto my tongue letting it slide down the right hole very slowly and carefully, a mistake now was going to hurt like hell and wake up half of the ward as I attempted to cough myself to death.

We managed to drink not one but two cartons of the milk shake but it took more than two hours and how she managed to hold the cartons still in front of me for all of that time amazes me today, her arms must have been screaming at her but she did neither rush me nor complain, not once.

Come morning I was in a position to whisper to my assailant, the anaesthetist, that I had eaten during the night and if he would like to leave my tablets with me, I will, in the fullness of time, eat those as well, I did struggle but managed them in the end, all crushed up and in tiny pieces, with a lot of milk and help from Linda.

I was now starting to get some feeling back and could move both legs and my hands about now though couldn't hold anything yet, not unless I wanted to spill or drop it.

I had little or no control over any of my muscles for quite some time, I couldn't support my weight or push myself up or little else to be honest.

I would constantly slide down the bed and have to ask for help to get back up and semi comfortable again, asking for help being the time consumer here. I was like a quadriplegic, my body malfunctioning, it was quite scary at times.

I am awake again, following my adventures with the toilet fairy I did apparently drop off for an hour or so, and feeling is coming back to my muscles, my skin, all of the bits and bobs especially those unwanted pain receptors and this, I am told, is good, I must be on the mend at last.

One more nasty session with the ventilator and associated drugs, it is so awful, I cannot bear to have my face touched like this, do not like things on my face at all especially near my damaged left eye.

I managed to complete the medicines and passed the test, I am on the mend at last and do not need to be in intensive care anymore.

Chapter seven

This morning it has been decided that I am to be put back on the main ward and I have a collection of ladies around me who are going to execute said task, I am as usual bloody terrified.

It is astounding how quickly one can get used to something, I was now getting used to being cut from head to foot, not being able to move and pissing through a pipe. I was not prepared to have this all changed again, I was as content as could be as every change involved more pain. Please, if only for a day or two, leave me alone.

I am disconnected from my plumbing; I now have only the pipe sticking out of my cock left to do as I have been temporarily disconnected from everything else in readiness for my transit away from cardiac intensive care.

The pipes that were hanging out of my tummy have been removed and stitched up now.

My attention is cleverly drawn by a nurse on my right speaking to me and as I look round the nurse on my left whips the pipe out of my cock complete with the attaching tape without even a by your leave sir, and when I yell and challenge her, rather squeak at her, she just advises me " trust me, it hurts a lot less if you do not know it is going to happen".

Oh well, something else out of the way but sadly I cannot feel my bladder and cannot at this time control my pee either so a bit of a wet bed is left behind me for someone else to clean up. Unusually for me, I am not feeling embarrassed about the wet bed, nor about my nakedness and my cock doing its level best to hide away, it is rather scared now, though it would be very hard to believe that this little frightened appendage has filled five prams.

I am far too concerned about the mammoth task ahead of me, it is no easy matter to find mobility when nothing will obey me, my body feels more like a cadaver, it feels as though it has been exhumed from the grave and stitched to my head, my head having enough trouble on its own.

Once completely disconnected from all of my pipes and sensors, I am brought a wheel chair for the transit to the next floor but unfortunately I am unable to get off of the bed and into it, I try but am completely unable to move myself towards the edge of the bed and when eventually do, with some assistance, get to the edge of the bed and elevate myself I am dizzy and unable to stand up or control my movements sufficiently to get into it, I cannot support myself or balance with my arms either, my hands being just as useless with so little feeling in my fingers and no feeling at all in my legs or feet. I feel more like a glove puppet than a man and wait for someone to shove their arm up my arse to control me.

It would be good to remember here that although I have lost quite a lot of weight, I am still at least twice as heavy as any of the staff around me and it takes quite a few hands to get me sorted out, support me and comfort me.

A person crane is brought over and I am bundled painfully into a cradle and hoisted up and into the waiting wheel chair like a bag of rubbish, I feel bloody awful, embarrassed, worried and really shaken by the experience.

I am taken at last with all of my belongings to the cardiac ward, the crane following behind like some awful praying mantis ready to pounce on me and do me harm.

The nurses are wonderful, as I lean forward my face lands against a rather large ladies bosom and when I ask if they can wait a minute because I am comfortable all have a good laugh and even the owner of the bosom strokes my hair in fun.

The reverse of getting out of the bed was equally or more problematic and painful and I was exhausted, wet with sweat and urine and not a little concerned as I was feeling so helpless that I could have wept. While in the cradle and suspended it proved impossible for me to breath, the cradle being flexible tightened around me squashing my chest as I was lifted and it really was bad, I would resist if told to do it again.

I needed the bed changing and I had been in it for exactly five minutes but no one complained to me or at me, everyone was good to me and I was soon asleep, plumbed back in to my anti biotic and insulin meters. I think Linda had turned up, cannot really remember though.

I now had to try and hold my bladder but unusually I couldn't feel my bladder, I couldn't feel my prostate or what ever bit stops you from peeing yourself, so couldn't squeeze it shut so to speak, the tap was not under my control so I took to using a bottle in the bed every half an hour or so until I thought I was getting the hang of it, the nurses must have thought me to be mad constantly having my hands under my blanket trying to take a pee but it was to turn out that I had suffered some irreparable damage in this area during the operation or the long sleep. To be honest, as I still couldn't feel my fingers properly it very much reminded me of those very early fumblings with young ladies who didn't know what to do with their thumbs.

I had a visit from Dave Wise and his wife.

Dave had still not been down for his operation yet but the real fun came from his wife when she said the wonderful statement " we all thought you were dead, you didn't come back to the ward like everyone else and none of us wanted to ask what had happened to you".

The date was 15th of December 2006 and I was hopefully on the mend though still feeling like shit with limited mobility, limited feeling and everything still smelling or tasting of anaesthetic.

Coughing was a major issue with everyone that had open heart surgery and until this moment it had been a case of grin and bear it. Part of the problem is that you are encouraged to cough, to bring up the phlegm that accumulates during the surgery and in my case much worse by lying still for more than a week, the trouble being that no one took the time to tell you how to safely cough.

Not here though, the ward sister paid far to much attention for that and she had perfected a way of constructing a pillow by wrapping up two towels in a pillow case which could then be hugged tight against the chest and hopefully help hold the sternum together reducing the amount of pain considerably especially if you had the time to get your arms crossed before the cough started.

This pillow was to become my very best friend for the next three months, it went everywhere with me, and was almost always within reach as coughing was to be constant and continuous, always very painful and sometimes quite scary, the only thing on this planet that could be more scary than a cough, was a sneeze, they were potentially lethal.

The pillow looked very much worse for wear because it hadn't been washed in three months, I wouldn't allow it just in case I needed it.

My nights were also to become rather scary now because every time I closed my eyes I would hallucinate, I would make up all sorts of images and locations, I could be any body, anywhere with no real rhythm or rhyme to it.

Because it was nearly Christmas the predominate theme was just that, Christmas, and my bed was a sleigh with me being dragged around the hospital at break neck speed, me yelling at the top of my voice for people to get out of the way or for people to hold my reindeer still.

The night staff recorded this and I was re visited by the anaesthetist, who examined me again and it was presumed that the cocktail of gases during surgery had either caused some damage to me or had lingered and was still in my system, either way, I was feeding those reindeer for nearly two weeks, it was as mad as galloping Shergar around Atlantis with Elvis and Lord Lucan in tow.

I was naming the reindeer, talking to them and truly believed them to be there in front of me, if I opened my eyes they were gone though.

I thought I had gone as mad as the people on the seventh floor and asked about rejoining them, how bad is that, I could go to the seventh floor and be completely barking mad all night long, calling out, yelling and being very very annoying, revenge, how sweet would that be.

Linda had kept up my supply of goodies and food, and my special supply of white powder which could be traded for good will if nothing else, even the nursing staff were coming to me to top up their own supplies when on a midnight pig out, this not being an unusual happening, I would often wake, being right next to the nursing station, to the smell of oriental food that had been delivered to the ward by a take away restaurant in Oxford.

I was myself getting a good selection of food stuffs but couldn't face eating anything, my throat was very sore, I was never sure where the food or drink would end up and cause coughing fits, which believe me were best avoided or it all just tasted of anaesthetic still .

I had by now lost nearly three stone in weight and the doctors were expressing concern for my lack of appetite, so much so that the food trolley would stop next to my bed and I could select anything that took my fancy, not just what I had pre ordered the day before, I had an absolute glut of jelly, ice cream, soft fruit and yoghurts. The nursing staff, were now monitoring what I was eating, calorie counting for the doctors, weighing me every day and the data went onto my notes.

This would continue for quite a few weeks to come even after I had returned home, I couldn't even eat my Christmas dinner. Sadly, I was to get my appetite back and would put on all the weight that I had lost, in the main due to my immobility created by my very sore right ankle and tired knee joints.

The next great adventure came when I needed to go to the toilet again, I had not been now for three days and would not use a bed pan but day shift on this ward had a glut of male nurses from the Philippines, they were all friendly and very helpful so I asked the question and yes was the response, they would unplug me from my machines and help me to the bathroom.

This nurse, whose name completely escapes me, though I do recall it being completely un pronounceable, asked if I would like to have a bath, my wounds were for the most part closed up and he thought the warm water would help my mobility issues, possibly get some feeling back to my extremities due to the changes of temperature against my skin.

He got a wheel chair from the corridor, helped me off of the bed and wheeled me, without my pipes and wires, into the bathroom where they had a crane to help get me into and out of the bath and even could be used for some support to aid getting on and off of the toilet.

He undressed me, just pants and a gown and while the bath was running he stood outside so that I could take a dump, oh boy was that good even if my bum cheeks and crack were still suffering with bed sores, I did have a lot of trouble doing the obvious clean up though, my hand felt like it belonged to a stranger, I could not hold toilet paper and it was a real struggle.

I wonder if I had been rude to anyone while I was in my extended sleep and they had taken to wiping my backside with sand paper, it was that sore now or in reality, was it how I had been given my tablets ?.

I called the nurse and he got me into this wind up crane, cursing my weight he managed to hoist me over the bath, winding the handle round and round like an insane dervish, swing round and down we go into foaming warm water, not allowed hot in here, it doesn't even come out of the taps hot just in case.

I had to stay sitting on crane chair while in the bath, to aid getting me back out should an emergency occur, it wasn't terribly comfortable but hey ho, I was in the bath.

The nurse washed my hair and my back, his mate, hopefully he was another nurse, came in and very carefully did my legs and I washed my private bits as best I could, I wasn't allowed to get my canulars wet or the dressings would come off, but it was good, it was like my first ever bath all over again, I cannot explain to you how wonderful it felt..

I suddenly had a very strange feeling that I had been here before, my first batch of déjà vu since entering the hospital complex, I began to remember the bathroom, pink wall tiles and grey vinyl flooring, suddenly my head was filled with memories of my days before the surgery, I was overjoyed with this collection of memories, I didn't feel so hollow as when I couldn't recall what had happened to me, I remembered meeting Dave Wise, his funny little wife, the staff and the loonies.

I was hoisted out of the water in better condition than I went in, I could remember lots of things including my home, my family and I wanted to get out of this place now, wanted to see home and my family urgently now, wanted to hug my young children, the older ones as well for that matter. I hadn't had the chance to really miss anyone because I hadn't remembered anyone until now.

I was aware that my family would have been missing me, worried for me and my selfish crusade on infection would make this worse for them, they would however, be aware that I was on the mend, Linda had kept up a news bulletin throughout my stay.

I was dried off and dressed for the first time in my own clothes, tee shirt and bed shorts, I felt so clean and chuffed with the memories and once wheeled back to bed I telephoned Linda to tell her what had happened, just a quick call because the nurses were hovering around me waiting to plumb me back into my pipes, insulin and anti biotic medicines though I managed to get out of wearing the ECG tabs, the oxygen monitor or the blood pressure cuff all of which had been on permanently for some ten days now and had left red wheals on my arms.

It was now so much less uncomfortable to lay down, obviously I had to stay on my back only, but more comfortable and easier to move about now without all of the monitors on and less of a worry about pulling on this wire or that pipe setting off alarms.

This lifted my mood as it also told me that the staff thought that I was on the mend and didn't need the constant monitoring though they did keep me next to the nurses station throughout my stay, maybe they knew that I could be trouble.

Chapter eight

I had a visitor today, my step brother Gary had come and found me and I was really pleased to see him, he is the son of my mums second husband John, who is such a lovely chap and we are all very fond of him.

Gary, like me, is a motorcyclist and it was good to hear about his journeys into Europe to see his Belgium girl friend, good to hear about his work etc.

Gary stayed for half an hour or so and then went off to work, he would later report to my mum and John what he had seen as he spoke to them most days.

I had refused all visitors other than my Linda because I am waging my own personal war on contamination / cross infection / dirt brought into the hospital completely unnecessarily and totally avoidable, so I denied my whole family including my children access to me until such time as I was home, I also didn't want the bother of making myself presentable to visitors.

I cannot understand the possible point of washing your hands or using the hand rub gels when you have just travelled into work on public transport and proceed about your duties in the same clothes, I have seen nurses and doctors entering and leaving the hospital in the clothes they work in all day, you could walk the dog, tread in dog piss and walk it straight onto the ward because they wear the same shoes, it is absolutely stupid.

I believe staff should wash and change into fresh uniforms every time they come on duty and it should be the NHS problem to provide said clean laundry, this would eliminate this issue, they should also change foot wear.

It was good to see Gary though, we have never been close and it was so good of him to come in and have a short chat.

The day to day goings on are quite interesting in themselves and normally happen as follows.

We would be woken quite early in the mornings, usually around half past six so that we could have tablets and injections as required. I have always found this routine to be a bit too rigid as it wouldn't hurt to leave you sleeping for half an hour or so longer, they cannot deal with everyone at once so why not deal with people as they wake.

This would be followed by ones ablutions' in the bathrooms if you were mobile and a bowl of warm water brought to you if you were not, though being not was no fun because personally I find trying to wash etc in bed rather difficult even if you have control of your hands, mostly I got washed though always had to do my bits and pieces myself.

I remembered when I had been in another hospital, a private patient, following surgery to my broken ankle. The staff nurse had brought me my requested and pre ordered sandwiches, fresh and hand made, not premade and wrapped in film, and a cup of tea when she politely asked me if there was anything else that she could do for me.

I asked her, very tongue in cheek, if I could have couple of young Philippine nurses to give me a good wash to remove the blood and bits from my leg, she said " two young Philippine nurses coming up" and sent me, true to her word exactly that except they were both men, she laughingly reminded me later that I had failed to specify a sex. Oh well, it was worth it if it brightened some ones day.

Breakfast would follow which normally involved some Eastern European asking you what you would like for breakfast followed very quickly by "we have Cornflakes or toast", why bloody well ask what I would like, and this would be escorted by a cup of tea or coffee, both of which could be either, they tasted the same to me. I would not be at all surprised to hear that they managed to give tea to the entire ward from just a single tea bag, it was so weak.

The nurses would then chase around making tidy for the ward rounds with the ward sister and all of the big chiefs, surgeons, consultants etc who would stop at each bed, call you a cabbage or similar and move on leaving me wondering what was just said. They seem to speak in code or Klingon with only their contemporaries understanding what they are saying, and that is when they are actually addressing you. I always made a habit of asking the nurses what the consultants had just said later on.

It would then be a rest time, peace would resume throughout the ward with the usual people going to or returning from surgery, drips and things topped up or emptied, insulin adjusted and any dressings sorted out.

The ward would then be descended on by an army of cleaners, mopping, dusting, polishing throughout, generally the cardiac units always appear much cleaner than everywhere else that I have visited in the hospitals, maybe they have more importance due to the very large contingent of consultants, surgeons and doctors.

Sadly though, I never did see anyone clean in a corner, always a huge great mop or broom pushing it all around, never cleaning it all up.

The day would progress slowly and before you knew it they would be bringing round the lunch, around twelve thirty normally.

Lunch would consist of something made from a mixture of dead animal and dead vegetable, always smelling and tasting the same, probably made from the same pot with different vegetables or pasta or rice etc.

I do believe that the chef was a master of his trade, it was like Les Dawson playing the piano, it takes a genius to be that bad, it was an art form and this chef was a master of his art and while I am aware of his remit, ie, budget per cover and content, no salt or butter products, it was still painfully and universally bloody awful.

Lunch would be cleared away and there was always a lot of uneaten food which in itself speaks volumes, pudding normally being the only reliable source of nutrition, a cup of tea or coffee again and that was it, the highlight of the day gone.

There was normally an enforced sleep period for a couple of hours each afternoon with curtains pulled around and absolutely no visitors allowed.

This was a good time to have a kip because for some unknown reason most of us seemed to find the long nights a painful and restless time, pain killers being in very short supply I might add though they would dish out the odd sleeping tablet or two. I was often quoted the adage that there should already be enough pain killers inserted when the operation was closing up, I shouldn't really be in need any additional pain relief.

Bugger me, that is one hell of a universal undertaking that we will all require the same amount of pain relief, wrong, again…

We would be woken by the curtains all being swished back and one could be confronted by the physio, the pharmacist, the diabetes nurse or even the priest, which is bloody scary I might add but time ticked by, book reading or quietly watching the silly little television which each bed had, very expensive and not comfortable at all to use with head phones on, I could never quite get the angle right to view while lying down.

There was a visiting period in the afternoons which went through to the evening, normally at its busiest when you were trying to eat some tea.

But always good to see Linda who usually turned up round meal times as well, normally armed with some goodies or other that I could manage to get down me, more jelly, fruit and ice cream, some soft cake or other.

Linda had got very much into the spirit of Christmas by now and decided to decorate my drug trolley and did one the same for Dave Wise.

She got paper plates and dressed them with beards and faces and fixed them to the top of the wheeled trolleys surrounded by tinsel, they were so good that they became our new best friends, remember, they had to go everywhere that we went because we were so attached to them, literally, and were a really big hit with the nursing staff and reminded me of the film Castaway, where the chaps best friend was a painted football that he called Wilson.

Linda did of course have to play the part of the laundry fairy as well, always something to take home and turn around, she was always amazed by how much laundry I could get through while doing nothing, it is difficult to eat loose, wobbly foods while lying down.

I am still not able to eat solid food and a lot of what Linda brings me is being eaten by the nursing staff or just thrown away, especially chocolate products, I always tried to have an open box for the staff on my locker.

I am existing on yoghurt, jelly and ice cream with the occasional cup of soup

Linda had today, brought in some Kentucky Fried Chicken which we sat down to eat in the visitors area but sadly it still tasted of anaesthetic and I still cannot swallow much so it all goes in the bin but bless her cotton socks for trying so hard.

I have been told off by the ward sister after I was found wandering around on the floor above with my trolleys in tow and only wearing a pair of pants and a tee shirt, I have no idea how I got there or why but think it is because I cannot remember going into the hospital and I have started looking for prompts and clues to try and kick start my memory, without success I might add, either way I am grounded and spied on a lot now to make sure I stay in my bed or chair, I think I may be a nuisance now.

The nightmares continue, I am still Father Christmas every night, still following a bunch of incontinent Reindeer through the hospital every time that I close my eyes, and apparently still calling out for someone to hold the reindeer while I feed them or deliver some presents, I also hear disco music and fantasize about going to a disco and water, there is a huge pool or lake in the middle of the complex which is full of sharks and dead people, I think I may be going bonkers. I ask the nurse how many people die here, how many patients do not make it through the surgery and she tells me none, not one person has died from the surgery for as long as she can remember, she tells me that they all die from food poisoning, cheeky bugger.

It is getting very close to Christmas and I am really starting to get depressed, I have been here now for six weeks and have had quite enough.

I am starting to feel well enough to go home, I can walk around the ward unassisted now, feed and drink on my own, within the limitations of a damaged throat, and with Linda's help I feel I could get in and out of bed, to the bathroom and even down the stairs to watch the telly, Linda had at this time stopped coming everyday, at the beginning she had been coming twice a day but the novelty had most definitely worn off and she was now worn out by it all, bless her.

I have made up my mind to make it my mission to get out of this place and hopefully the reindeer will not follow me home.

The next day I get a visit from the Indian consultant who works on professor Taggarts team, his name also eludes me but I remember having conversations with him when I first woke up in intensive care.

He is a round faced, round bellied jolly fellow, laughing and smiling all of the time and it is a pleasure to engage with him if only for a short while.

He checked me over and read my notes and proclaimed that I should be able to go home in a week or two, I was not at all happy with this statement and asked why when people were coming and going all of the time around me.

He said " You have had a huge amount of work done to your heart, you have been asleep for a very long time, you have a chest infection and you are diabetic, requiring insulin, and you have such a huge chest and very long arms which worries me, you could pull your chest apart quite easily and I want you to stay here for a bit longer until we are sure that you are well enough".

There would be a time to come soon when I wished that I had listened to him, his was the voice of reason and he would prove to be correct for I was to damage my chest going back to work too soon and have never been well.

I was not best pleased with this news, I was sure that I would get better so much quicker at home and Linda was now showing signs of stress, tiredness and I was worried about her doing all of these journeys, rushing around shopping for me and taking messages at home, I was also very worried, and it was to prove rightly so, about my business for my brother was running things in my absence and making a prize cock up of it all.

He had in fact taken over the company, elevating himself to managing director and as far as he was aware sole owner even though in reality he owned nothing, he was gutted and said so when I didn't die and actually managed to get back to work, sadly too late to save the business, he had spent all the money and ruined everything.

The only up side was that because he had made legal claim to everything, including all of the shares, when it came time to call in the receiver he alone had to carry the can and although he did his best to implicate me in the failings, was make bankrupt, ha ha thieving bastard, I was free to start over again with the same clients and workforce but a shame that he had robbed me of my money and vehicles.

I must admit to missing him though, he is still my brother but there is no going back now, his ownership and elevated position of what was my business and my down fall and not dying as he had wanted cannot ever be put behind us. He had put nothing into the company, not money, vehicles, staff or customers, yet laid claim to all.

When Stuart had been ill, I had been back and forth to Dorset to visit him in the hospital, though I was in hospital and off work for fourteen weeks or so and very much at deaths door, he didn't so much as telephone let alone pay me a visit, arsehole.

I have not seen or spoken to any friends or family since coming here so Linda had been keeping everyone informed of my progress, apart from my gym training partner who made the effort to track me down when I hadn't spoken to him for a couple of weeks, Mark Woodley, bless him, his smiling face did pick me up.

Mark and I had a pact when out at the gym, usually playing squash followed by a sauna, followed by a pint or two of beer.

My insurance didn't cover me for sport so if I became ill playing squash, he was to drag me off the court and up to the bar before calling for any help otherwise they wouldn't pay out. Mark and I used to see who would get to go the reddest, we were both over weight and played far too hard.

He stayed an hour or so, good to see him, good to chat though if I am honest, there was an awful lot that I didn't remember still and spent a lot of time agreeing with him, sorry Mark.

My mum called me at the hospital this evening, I must confess to getting rather choked up and could hear her doing the same at the other end of the telephone, she would be suffering this in her own way, thinking about my dad and what had happened.

She told me off for not looking after myself better and it was lovely to have that normality, she always told me off.

I promised to make the trip down to Dorset where they had retired to as soon as I was well enough to drive and had completed my eight week statute driving ban, my post heart surgery ban that everyone automatically gets. I was so looking forward to a cuddle from her.

I discussed the position regarding staying in the hospital longer with Linda that evening when she came to see me, with some grub, she was crestfallen, I could see it on her face even when she didn't comment.

We only live thirty minutes from the hospital and did feel that we could manage my recovery better from home and decided to move in that direction, I made it quite clear to her that if she took me out of here, she would have to look after me.

My wounds seemed to be healing, I had got the hang of coughing now, and I could use an ordinary bathroom and everything else Linda was there to help me with, dressing was very difficult as I couldn't even put socks on yet and definitely couldn't feel to do up buttons or zippers, washing was also going to be a problem with getting in or out of the bath extremely difficult, if not impossible, Linda was still at this point shaving me as well.

We were to get the hang of getting in and out of the bath, I do not like taking a shower as most shower heads seem level with my face and I have to bend to get beneath them.

I would back up to the ready run bath and sit on the side, sliding my bum into the water leaving my legs over the side and Linda would wash me, progressing to using this method to get in or out but turning round to sit normally during my lazy soaks. In this way, all I had to do to get out was progressively slide more and more of my rather heavy legs over the side as Linda pulled me by my arms, bloody painful none the less and most definitely put off until really needed each week.

The following day I asked if I could see the Indian consultant or Prof Taggart again so that I could discuss going home and obviously was told that it would be a long wait but they would see what they could do, I understood this because they were always very busy men.

I discussed the possibility of coming off of the insulin and onto tablets, coming off of the anti biotic liquid and again converting this to a tablet.

The problems raised by nursing staff were huge, though I felt not insurmountable, and very valid from their point of view, everyone was trying to make me stay at this point.

Because I was eating no solids they felt insulin to be the best way of controlling the diabetes and that going on to tablets meant having my control doses in lumps ie two or three times a day rather than constantly dripping into my system, the machine delivering my antibiotic doses was doing the same, supplying a constant measured dose twenty four hours a day and yes tablets could be substituted but not as well and I would run the risk of taking them without food in my stomach, I was already at this time taking six other tablets a day plus pain relief so a few more wouldn't hurt, surely.

The above conversation was reinforced when the cardiac consultant paid me a very brief visit late that evening but I had become more determined than ever now, how silly was I, he was to be proven correct in his diagnosis of my future.

The following day after breakfast I was feeling very low and in a fit of pique pulled out my pipes and needles and insisted that I wanted tablets from now on and that today Elvis, the white powder man, would be leaving the building, quite bold of me really because not only did I not know where I was, I didn't have a clue how to get out of there.

Hoist by my own petard, they would say if they knew what it meant.

After lots of attempts to placate me the pharmacist was called, the doctor wrote up the prescriptions and I had to spend some time with the physiotherapists who had to confirm that I could walk and climb stairs safely.

They helped me to get dressed, all the while telling me how silly I was being and what difference could a few more days make and trotted me up and down the ward which I thought went rather well though as I hadn't had to move more than twenty or thirty feet for quite a few weeks was painfully obvious to them that I was struggling.

We then had to tackle a stair case which was fortunately very close to my bed so once we had gone up one very slow and shaky flight and back down again I was able to collapse on my bed and sleep for some hours, I was that knackered but the physio had passed me off as safe, if rather stupid and she probably thought me to be ignorant and arrogant not listening to the advise on offer.

My wounds were dressed, especially the ones on my arms where I had removed the needles (canulars) myself, which obviously got me a telling off but I had to get the attention of the right people or I was not going to get my way, I was at this time also thankful that my mum was not about as she would have given me a right telling off and probably a smack or two for behaving so badly.

It is rather amusing really that the smacks from my five foot nothing mother stopped hurting when I was about fourteen yet she would still dish them out hurting no one but herself.

When Linda came to see me I was pipe and cable free, sat in shorts and tee shirt beaming with pleasure and trying to eat and drink as much of the produce around me rather than have to throw it all into the bin, I supposed that it would be a lot easier to carry if it were in my tummy.

I told her that I would be going home in an hour or so, once all of my paperwork was completed and my medicines were ready from the pharmacy.

She busied herself by going too and fro from the car shuttling the huge collection of books, shavers, clothing and paraphernalia associated with a long stay away from home and after a couple of trips we were all ready to get on our way.

The next task was to get me dressed, not for the first time, she had to put my socks on for me, hold my trousers while I stepped into them, put my shoes on and lace them up, then take off my tee shirt, put a shirt on me, do up all of the buttons and finally help me to tuck myself in and do up my belt, my trousers now being two or three sizes to big as I was three stone lighter than when I came in to hospital.

The look on her face was mixed, a bit of thank god we are getting out of here and quite a bit of how am I going to manage, he is so bloody useless, bordering on being a spastic.

Paper work was exchanged, medicines packaged away and good byes all round, they had all been really good to me but I am just passing through to them, no tears, just a job.

I often think of them, can still see some of the faces, still remember the good and less good times spent on the cardiac ward, I am not keen to go back though.

Chapter nine

I didn't think I would need a wheel chair or anything so off we went, the trip home had begun and I think Robert Falcon Scott had an easier time walking to the South Pole than I had getting to that bloody car park, it was all of three hundred yards away, three hundred very big yards.

The most obvious thing was the wearing of shoes, I had had nothing on my feet for so long that it had become completely alien to me and I was feeling really uncomfortable even though Linda had cleverly selected my soft and comfortable boat shoes and cotton socks.

The wounds between my legs especially the huge cut right into my left groin was rubbing as I walked so I had to walk really slowly and walk like I had something unspeakable in my pants, the ends of the un dissolved stitches sticking out like the feathers in a down pillow each feeling like a needle.

Normally when I walk this corridor I am amazed by the humanity, the cosmopolitan diversity of mankind, people of different colours and creeds, religions and ethnisticity and the staggering amount of people that throng these area's mostly though I look at the woman's institute cafe stall and fancy a liver sausage roll, this time however I didn't, the noise was almost unbearable, the pushing and shoving, tooing and froing was most unwanted and I couldn't wait to get out of there, away from the doings of mankind and back to the peaceful seclusion that I had become so used to. I was already missing my bed in the cardiac ward.

I was unable to carry anything, it was now December but I couldn't even manage to carry my own coat and had to stop every thirty yards or so, a trip that would normally be walked in three or four minutes took as much as twenty minutes and in the end Linda sat me down near to the main entry / exit doors and went off on her own to collect the car and bring it much closer to the doors reducing my final trip, by this time I was soaked in sweat and rather unwell.

Linda had only a small Toyota at this time and never before had it felt so small, she should by rights have brought my car which is much larger but that was the very reason why she didn't drive it, I wished she had as it hurt so much to fold myself into the front seat and although I was trying to be really brave in case she changed her mind and took me back, I don't think I looked very brave.

By rights I should have been enjoying the freedom, the release from my hospital prison, but I was not, I was quite worried about things going wrong, rather anxious about Linda being able to cope.

The journey home was terrible, Linda being a timid driver has a tendency to hug the kerb hitting every single drain or gully cover and as the roads around Oxford are not the best it was a very long and painful trip for me obviously made much worse by my injuries, and not entirely Linda's bad driving but I vowed there and then that she would get a bigger car, a lot bigger with some suspension, if I had my way.

It was nice to be in the open again, the sun wash shining down even though it was the nineteenth of December, nice to look upon the world again, the trees had lost a lot more leaf since I last saw them, the roads were a mucky colour as they has been gritted since I last saw them.

We eventually arrived home and I had to get out of the car and into the warmth as quick as I could if I was not to catch a cold, getting out of the car being the biggest and hardest hurdle to date I think.

Linda got on with the business of emptying the boot and back seat of the car while I just sat and pondered my situation, I didn't know how to get out of the car, couldn't for the life of me think how, given the state of my arms and legs and the nausea that I was now suffering, how I would ever get out of this horrendous little car, indeed, I wasn't sure that I even wanted to.

For some strange reason I wasn't pleased to be here, I was now quite frightened about being here and if I got out of the car, there would be no going back.

I the end Linda came round to my side and helped me unfold myself, helping me lift one leg at a time out of the car, helping me to my feet and guiding me along the front path to the door taking great care with the three little steps that catch a few people out.

As Linda opened the front door and I walked inside my emotions finally got the better of me and I exploded into a blubbering mess, I cried my heart out, I had never expected to get home, didn't expect to survive the surgery and I was feeling rather sorry for myself, needing a nice cup of tea.

I was home, I had been away for thirty seven days and I was home.

I was now completely knackered and had to find enough energy to climb the stairs, I really was on my last legs and once Linda had removed my shoes I climbed Everest for the first time, no oxygen either, well blow me down, Linda had not been idle while I had been away and the bed room was decorated and had a nice new remote slim line TV with digital viewing package in the bedroom, the furniture that we had bought before I was ill had been delivered and the whole bedroom looked very welcoming indeed with big fluffy pillows and cushions, new curtains and carpet.

There sat on the pillows was my favourite teddy bear, I had completely forgotten about him until now, I grabbed hold of him as Linda undressed me and folded my sorry self softly into the bed, big fluffy duvet and I was soon fast asleep .

I very soon came to realise the benefits of hospital beds because if the back of the bed is raised mechanically, I would not have to sit up using my stomach muscles which are in turn attached to my rather sore abdomen and chest. It had proven impossible to lie on my side, far to much effort too get there and far to much pain once I had achieved it.

I could only lie on my back, semi propped up with several million pillows, all of which within ten minutes of getting comfortable would desert me, deflate and become useless and as such impossible to rest for long.

Linda, bless her, would no sooner get me settled and leave the room and I would be so uncomfortable again that rather than call her I would have to struggle and sort myself out, even the act of rotating enough to pick up the supplied cup of tea from the bed side cabinet was enough for me to leave it there to get cold, even turning my head and neck was uncomfortable if not damn right painful and was to be avoided. This wasn't helping because I cannot turn my eyes very much due to the amount of surgery to my left eye so I found it rather difficult to look at people when they spoke to me.

My enemy number one was coughing, something that happened quite frequently as my body fought to get rid of the anaesthetic that lingers in the lungs and also the build up of fluid that happens if you lay still for a long time and I had been doing that for a very long time now.

Enemy number two was most definitely the sneeze, I would just be thinking that my chest was starting to join and settling down nicely when I would sneeze and upset the applecart, I would sneeze with the most dreadful violence, not a little a-tissue but a full on sneeze that is both violent and very noisy, the result being a very sore chest.

Quite often I would have a run of half a dozen or so of these mega sneezes ending up with me in agony and tears rolling don my cheeks and not just a little bit scared about my chest bone join. We will not discuss sneezing when both hands are used to hold your chest still, arms crossed and squeezing tight, the snot goes every where, as you can imagine.

That evening I did just stay in bed and because of the way that I had to sleep, ie propped up on my back, Linda had no choice but to relocate to the front bedroom, doors open in case I needed her in the night.

Strangely I didn't actually bring the reindeer home with me, I never saw them again which is a blessing really because I had run out of food for them and with Christmas day only just around the corner I feel sure Santa needed them back.

I was however really pleased to get my teddy bear back, I had really missed him and he was good company for me while alone in bed, this you may feel to be rather unusual for a big rough tough guy but, when I split with my last wife, my little girl, when she came to stay with me at weekends, always put a teddy into bed with me, so that I wouldn't be alone at night, she didn't realise that I was never alone at night, I was internet dating and shagging my brains out, but the habit of the bear stuck, so much so that if the bear falls onto the floor at night I will wake and retrieve him, if the missus got out of bed I would be none the wiser.

It was nice to have the digital box on the television because there was something on 24/7 so if awake in the night I could watch something and quite often I found it easier to fall asleep to some kind of background noise

I could hear Linda snoring away so I knew that she wasn't suffering too much being displaced to the front bedroom and she would often bring me drinks as and when needed.

It is quite appalling what crap is on day time TV, I had little else to do other than watch TV or sleep as holding a book comfortably was still a few weeks off, there is only so much you can stand.

The following morning was difficult, I needed to pee and it was becoming increasingly urgent, it couldn't be put off any longer and I called Linda to give me a hand, I was feeling rather groggy and not at all steady on my feet when I finally managed to get out of bed, this taking at least five minutes just to get from lying position to a seated one and wet with sweat as a result of so much exercise. This was also day one on the new tablets for both my diabetes and the anti biotic for the chest infection not least the new blood pressure tablets, beta blockers, blood thinners, aspirin, ulcer busting drugs as well as a couple of nitrates to deter further heart attacks and I was also taking pain killers, so I was understandably feeling very much under the weather, my blood sugar level was out of measure and I was feeling sick.

All this grief just to take a piss.

Peeing had become a bit of an issue because I had become unable to do it standing up which obviously meant as we had no pee bottles at home, which I had now been used to for some weeks, I had to try and sit on the toilet.

This you might think is a very normal thing to do but in my case it was an extraordinary problem, I was very sore, my groin wounds were now starting to swell up and getting rather puffy, my bum crack still hadn't healed completely, I have a sneaky suspicion that they were abusing me while I was asleep in recovery unit or the nurse who was wiping my bum needed her nails cutting.

Also, I wasn't entirely sure what I was sitting on due to a lack of feeling, so it was quite possible for me to put weight down on my testicles, I would feel it then.

It appears that I cannot feel my bladder and not a great deal of feeling in my cock either, something was wrong but we would give it plenty of time before humiliating myself in front of my GP or back at the hospital. I rather like my GP and didn't want to disgrace myself by revealing that I suffered from a Pigmy cock.

I had to sit and wait, I could not squeeze to make myself go and only a little patience and gravity would make it happen, it sometimes took me more than half an hour to do it into a bottle and looking back it seemed like a good deal of my time was spent holding my cock because I think I was going every hour rather than risk a wet bed.

I was also quite a few days without a bowel movement, charming this is not but quite a problem to me, again a lack of feeling until it became just too late and I had far too much feeling, I was in dreadful pain and in serious danger of exploding and redecorating the bathroom walls to match the new chocolate brown towels that Linda had bought, in my absence.

I was fortunate throughout this entire time that I neither pooped nor peed myself at all, I do not know how I could have dealt with the embarrassment if Linda had had to clear up after me, or worse, clean me up as well.

Linda managed to get me to the bathroom and helped me on to the pan but I just couldn't go, I needed urgently to do it but just couldn't and in the end couldn't get back to the bed room either, I had become utterly exhausted just getting to the bathroom, you would have thought from all the fuss that I was using the one next door, no, it was only twelve feet away but still as much as I could manage.

Linda called her son in law Kevin, to come round and help me back to the bed, I was completely exhausted, covered in sweat from head to foot and getting quite desperate, it would have to happen soon or I would need help, but he did manage to get me back to bed though I couldn't sit, I needed to get off of my bottom and almost threw myself at the bed flat on my back.

Linda called her daughter Rachael now and asked her to pop into Boots the chemist and pick up some sort of suppository, God alone knows how I would insert them as my fingers were useless and I could hardly reach round there anyway, Linda bless her had already volunteered, fortunately that was enough to encourage me back to the bathroom and with one almighty effort and a huge push it was all over bar the paperwork, so to speak, I really must write and apologise to the people at the water treatment works, sorry for that.

I was now exhausted and quite annoyed with myself for believing that I was ready to be at home, I now knew that I was not, that I should still be in the hospital being looked after.

The above bathroom tales are a hugely important part of this tale because it helps to indicate the level of hopelessness that you fall into when your mobility suffers such a huge setback and how dependant and reliant one has to become on partners or worse, strangers.

I was now so tired that I had to have another cup of tea and an extended sleep, I slept so deeply that I awoke in an absolute panic yelling my head off for help because I had rolled over in my sleep and was now lying face down, on my chest and couldn't summon either the knowledge or the courage to turn back over, in the end I had to slide out of the bed onto my knees, sit up onto the edge of the bed with Linda heaving with all of her tiny might, and restart all over again, the right way up, what an adventure, what a fright.

I do not want to be doing that again in a hurry.

That evening, the first for many weeks I had visitors, I got to see Rachael and Kevin again but this time with their little boy, Linda's grandson, Lewis who I am incredibly fond of and I think he quite likes me.

I like to think myself a grandfather to him as his real grandfather is sadly missing from the scene most of the time and quite frankly, I do object when he does turn up, seemingly in glory, though I keep that to myself.

I then had the good fortune to have my middle son Tom, 26 years old now, pay me a visit which happens very much less than I would prefer because he is a loving lad, big like me, honest and a professional chef but working up in York which is two hundred miles away, with him was my future daughter in law, yes you guessed it, Rachael, we have three in the family now.

He was passing by, having visited his mum and I was really pleased to get a hug from him, he is six feet five inches tall and eighteen stones in weight but still likes his cuddles from his dad, he was shocked to see the skinny me, or shall we say slightly less me, covered in these horrendous wounds.

Last but not least, my ex wife brought the two youngest of my children to see me, though she is strictly up to the front door only, not allowed in.

I have looked forward to this moment for a long time, they are only 12 and 10 years old and have been very worried about me and although they still find me on my back at least I am breathing and can have a cuddle or two though Joshua, always inquisitive, was feeling rather cheated at not being able to see what the ward and theatres were like inside.

The above activity quickly wears me out and Linda feeds me, waters me, and gets me back off to bed, where I am soon fast asleep again.

Linda is a very adventurous cook, really good stuff that still tasted awful to me, I still had the anaesthetic taste in my mouth, nothing tasted right anymore and I was still losing weight, I did have the spare body mass though because I was still only just under twenty stone with my target weight something like eighteen to nineteen stone so no danger yet, it was just the amount of fibre and vitamins that would create ongoing issues especially in the bathroom departments.

A few days plodded past, I was getting better each day and spent more time either in the study writing or down stairs in the lounge watching TV or reading my stock of magazines.

Rehabilitation following surgery this extensive is a slow process, ups and downs; good days follow bad days, sleepless nights and coughing fits.

Sadly I have quite a lot of swellings and infections, three in my chest wound and five on my legs with the biggest being a lump the size of a golf ball right in my groin.

I had to keep these as clean and sterile as I could, Linda helping when needed but still wasn't getting on top of the problems and was becoming very sore and regretting my haste in leaving the hospital, not for the first time either.

The wound to my throat seems to be healing at last, I can swallow if careful, the wound to my neck had gone and the bed sores are definitely better, surprisingly so considering how long I am spending on my arse.

The wound that is taking some time to sort out is where they taped the breathing pipe while on life support which removed a lot of hair and skin from the back of my head and neck, this is still sore and I seem to be forever picking at it, very much to my beloveds annoyance, I wish I had bought shares in Savlon.

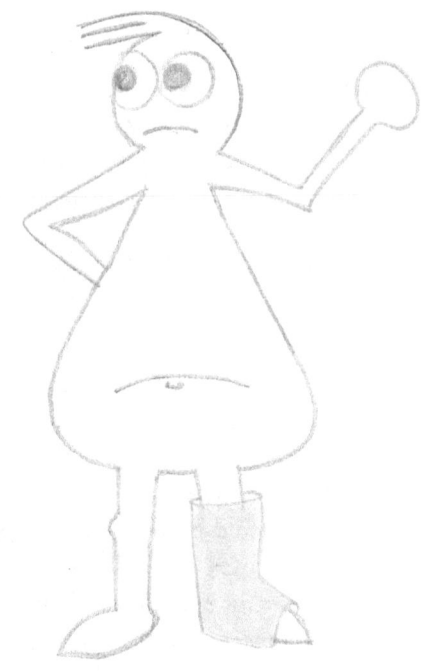

Chapter ten

Linda had arranged for us to spend Christmas day with her daughter and although I would very much have preferred to stay at home, I dutifully dressed, or was dressed, and suffered the short journey round to her house, only half a mile or so but still uncomfortable none the less especially the bloody awful task of getting in and out of the car again.

Embarrassingly for me, I have not been able to get Linda anything for Christmas, our first one together and I can do nothing about it, I have the money but just cannot get to a shop or ask others to do so because there just hasn't been enough time.

Rachael's husbands parents and brother are there for Christmas lunch as well as Lewis, my little mate.

Everyone seems pleased to see me, they are all very caring and kind, sitting me down out of harms way while dinner is prepared and drinks passed around, I was not drinking though.

I try very hard to eat some dinner but it is both tasteless to me and already quite cold by the time it is on the table so I eat nothing.

After the lunch I really need to lie down, everyone is going to be opening presents but I really cannot face it so Linda and Rachael tuck me up on Rachael's bed and I sleep for three or four hours while they all get on with their Christmas day, I am content to be out of the way, it is far better than the fuss and bother.

I am pleased when we get home; I have decided that I am not really ready to be out and about yet.

My daughter, also called Rachael pays me a visit; it is so nice to see her and her partner, Felix.

I haven't heard from my family since I got home and am quite pleased to get a phone call from my sister Sally and from my Mum and John as well.

Boxing Day is spent at home, peace and quiet at last though I am aware that Linda prefers a noisy family Noel, maybe she should have left me in the hospital until after Christmas

Linda had decided to go to her parents for New years Eve as we cannot go out to celebrate and we pack up and make the journey on the afternoon of the thirty first, last day of this extremely trying year in which I have been divorced, re married, separated and moved house three times in twelve months, changed my company twice, had major health problems and now it is at an end with the new one looking no better, bollocks, makes me feel that it isn't worth this constant struggle, this nagging pain and uselessness.

We arrive at Bill and Maureen's 120miles away, mid afternoon, rotten journey in Linda's little car because she still insists on driving in the gutter, me getting the jolt of every man hole cover or gully and following our quick hello's I am straight to bed and sleep the afternoon away with Linda waking me for dinner, nice, anaesthetic with anaesthetic for pudding, my favourite but we did have a tipple, me included as the clock swept past twelve.

The night was very difficult for me, with Linda sharing the same bed, something which had become unusual, my having to sit up all night and the increasing discomfort with my wounds, I was really starting to suffer now.

At two o'clock in the morning I could stand it no longer and woke Linda, we had to get me to a hospital because my wounds were weeping and the golf ball in my groin felt like it was now a grapefruit and I wasn't keen on grapefruit. Apparently, as an additional piece of information, grapefruit can react with some of my drugs and be quite fatal to me.

She dressed us both and we crept out and down into Worthing, West Sussex, only five miles from where we were staying, Linda finding the hospital by memory.

There was very little going on but despite the urgency that I explained my problem to be were kept waiting an hour before being seen, I had to keep wandering up and down because my groin hurt too much to sit.

The triage nurse took a careful look and then I had to wait about to be seen by a rather arrogant Indian doctor who issued me with a prescription for anti biotic tablets which in size were more suited to a horse, I didn't know whether to swallow them or just stick them up my arse, maybe he was in the know of what had been going on in Oxford.

The nurse came back in popped me onto the examination couch and carefully removed all of the stitches that had refused to dissolve, which, unbeknown to me, have been causing the infections as they had now started to rot and the smell was disgusting.

She then applied some special infection pads / dressings to each wound and cleaned me up, the grapefruit had luckily exploded without any residual damage to my testicles at this point, she also gave us a handful of spare pads to see out the next couple of days, it did however feel like I had pissed my self walking about with wet shorts on, puss not piss.

We stayed at Linda's, parents house until mid day of the new year and took a steady trot back home and nothing much happened over the next few days, steady progress was made in all departments, I could now wash and dress myself without too much help and had regained my appetite at last, the anaesthetic had finally worn off, I could even take a bigger breath which didn't rattle with fluid and I was now looking forward to getting back to work, I was bored.

It is quite a strange thing that while I was really poorly, I do not remember being bored but as soon as I started to get better, boredom became a major issue with discontent being a close second.

I hadn't driven my new car for more than a few miles since it was new, just weeks before I became ill, and was now really looking forward to getting out and about again, I honestly do really enjoy driving still, even after all of these years and all of the thousands of miles that I have done, I love everything automotive.

At last, eight weeks have now past and I am getting up at five in the morning and going off to work though in truth I very quickly realise just how difficult it is all going to be when I cannot tie my shoe laces or pull on some slip on shoes, Linda has to help again.

I have some sandwiches and a flask ready, you guessed it, Linda did it all again, I am dressed and I am willing.

I am also to discover how painful driving is, I cannot turn my head or shoulders to look round and have huge blind areas because of it.

I drive down to Kingston in surrey, a gentle trot and not too much traffic but struggle getting parked in the multi story car park, because I am so much later on site than I would usually be, the bottom ten levels of the car park are full and I have to go round and round and round and bloody round with each turn of the steering wheel hurting like hell, when I finally manage to find a space and finally get parked I am so completely knackered that I consider going straight back home, I don't though.

The walk from the car park to the site was only two or three hundred yards but it seemed to me more like a couple of miles, it took me over twenty minutes so it might as well have been, I arrived slightly moist and tired.

I have missed everybody on site, all of the sub contractors, my two younger brothers and am really quite pleased to see them all again, except for my stupid and arrogant brother Stuart who seems to be making a bloody pigs ear of everything and is very quick to assert his self found glory by starting an argument, I went home again.

I am not into stressful situations anymore, I have had years and years of this and my newly repaired heart doesn't react well to upset, neither do my kidneys or liver for that matter.

Within a week or two it becomes obvious that the fourteen weeks that I have been off of work have allowed Stuart and Sally to completely ruin the company, Stuart has not kept his eye on the ball, has been drugged up most of it with his new found cash cow and Sally didn't exercise the control that I thought she would, didn't want the rows with him either as with his drink and drug habits he is both aggressive and argumentative, even when completely wrong.

I have left the business and left Stuart to carry the can, he wanted my company so now he can go down with it, the stupid selfish twat.

On speaking to my clients, they were always my clients, Stuart was universally disliked because he thought too much of himself and not enough of the client, they were pleased he had made a cock up for himself, work was still on offer if I still wanted so I started again, this time with Billy as a co director and we just took over where Stuart had cocked up, even to the point of being paid for work that they had started.

At first I tried to work on the tools to help to get the business off the ground but I was not getting better as quick as I was led to believe I should, the rehabilitation nurses were also some what surprised with my lack of healing.

I should have rested far more than I did, I should have listened to the nursing staff and rehabilitation specialists, I should have believed that I wasn't ready to leave the hospital, I didn't and have been ill for a very long time.

I had started the rehabilitation program in an Oxford gymnasium, run by the Oxford group of hospitals and classes set up just for heart patients.

I am quite amazed to find that out of a class of twenty, I am the only open heart patient there, everyone else is either post heart attack or post stent so I am an interest to most.

I struggle to keep up with my work our program, I suppose it would be called a fitness program were I fit.

It is not long before I have to stop going due to ill health again and I do not get invited back, I am a risk.

Chapter eleven

I have collapsed at home a couple of times and Linda told me to get to the doctors if I can.

I had already had a letter from my own GP advising me that as I had moved away from their catchment area I had to enrol with a surgery closer to where I now lived in Thame, Oxon.

I was feeling pretty poorly when I got to my local surgery and I was stood in a queue to speak with the receptionist when she noted that I didn't look the right colour, I was drenched with sweat from head to foot and was close to collapse.

She called for assistance and all hell broke loose as a well rehearsed drill was brought into play and I was on a bed being attended to quicker than a quick thing, where I was quickly unconscious, nurses put needles in for fluids, and ECG appeared and so did my new doctor though I didn't know it at the time.

They were extremely professional, an ambulance had already been called and once stabilised I was soon dispatched back to the John Radcliffe, after having the dubious and embarrassing exit through the waiting room past all of the patients that I had so obviously kept waiting, I never did get to fill in the forms to enrol at this surgery.

Linda had to arrange to have my car collected from the surgery and brought back to the house, that worried me quite a lot because I do not like people driving my cars.

The ambulance people took ten minutes or so sorting me out in the car park before we started the plod over to the JR in Oxford, again.

As before, as soon as the heart word is used, I was rushed straight into triage and checked out, the ECG shows nothing and various doctors can hear nothing unusual, following chest X rays, and the morphine induced sleep while they once again take blood to check for tell tales which advise if I have had another heart trauma and at the end of the tests I am sent home with the unconfirmed guessed diagnosis that I have fluid around my heart which is not that unusual following heart surgery.

There was no evidence on which to base this discovery but at least it got me out of the A&E and confirmed that I wasn't at imminent risk and hadn't had a heart attack or similar, I was just unwell.

It was may 2007 and this was the start of the new health program called "lets guess what is wrong with Andrew" the main player being the heart consultant that they discussed my case with over the telephone who was so talented that he could diagnose down the phone line and because the attending doctor now had someone to fall back on to back him up, could put his chin out and declare what was wrong with me, sadly he was so terrible wrong.

I continued to ail, never getting any better, always in a lot of pain but at least I now have a doctor who takes me seriously, listens and cares about my predicament, even to the point of seriously annoying the cardiac team until she gets some answers and gets me seen, her name is Dr Meryl

Vaughan and she is thoroughly lovely, hugely talented and totally committed.

Within the week I have the symptoms again, I am stood in our hallway trying to put a jumper on over my head when I become stuck with the jumper neither on nor off, stuck half way but the pain in my chest is so great it knocks me to the floor, I cant move and I am lying across the front door so that it cannot be opened.

Linda has no option this time but to call the Ambulance again and they turn up, just after the fire brigade.

The paramedic has been fantastic as usual, he has run round to the back of the house where Linda has let him in though the gate and in through the rear French doors, he is now able to help me.

They get the jumper off and give me some oxygen and get me up and away from the front door, package me up as usual helping me into the waiting ambulance, down the three steps of the front garden.

Blow me down, I have just noticed that the fire engine is driven by a woman fire fighter, that's a turn up for the books; I bet she is good though.

Once stable again, ie drips in, morphine, anti sickness injections, oxygen and inside leg measurements taken we are again on our way, blue lights and sirens all the way back to Oxford, Linda in close company behind in her car, her new more comfortable car I might add because in the interval between hospital trips we had been out and purchased a nice Citroen C4 automatic fully loaded in metallic silver, whoopee.

This time, following the same tests and X-rays, blood letting etc they diagnose the problem as digestive issues or something unknown but could be a clot on my lung, who knows, they certainly didn't.

I have now had five emergency attendances at the JR A&E and my beloved is taking me back again, I can hardly stay conscious as I am in so much pain.

I have now developed a beautiful breast, right between the other two which while quite striking is not entirely welcome and I obviously have an infection in my chest wound or sternum and as this seems to be the same style of discomfort that I have had over the past few months feel that this is related, only as this time it is visual, bright red in fact, so the doctors may not need to guess so much .

Linda is not really satisfied with there explanations and she insists that I will not be going home until some thorough tests and examinations are carried out, she is at her whit's end and cannot continue with this not knowing what is wrong with me all of the time, she is also bored with making this journey.

I am admitted to the hospital at first to cardiac services and then once checked over and checked in, which takes most of the night, I am sent up stairs once again, this time the sixth floor which is as bad as the seventh floor menagerie.

I see people who tended to me when I stayed on the seventh floor all that time ago and I recall that Linda told me that they had come down to intensive care to visit me after my heart operation which is really quite sweet and apparently unique.

The following morning I am attended by two very attractive lady doctors
who's names I cannot remember and I sense something is going on because all of a sudden I am flavour of the month.

It is obvious that our protests the previous evening have not fallen on deaf ears and at last the hospital is about to treat me with the urgency that my extended illness is rightly due.

I am booked to go for every test known to man and after breakfast I am wheeled down for an MRI, X ray and CT scans, I also have an introduction to a liquid aural morphine " Oramorf" which along with the Morphine Sulphate tablets become my new best friends.

Upon my return I am quite unusually greeted again by these two doctors who explain to me that they have found the cause of all the pain and the swelling to my sternum, my chest has failed to join, I have a non union of my sternum so it is held together by the wires and my skin only which allows a lot of mobility in my chest coupled to a lot of discomfort and risk of associated infections.

That explains a lot of things, why I didn't like turning my shoulders or moving my arms above my head, why I couldn't look round, why I had a third tit, admittedly sans nipple.

The CT scan showed similar results, none of this could be seen by conventional X-ray machinery because there was a chewing gum like substance filling the crack so to all intense and purposes no gap would show.

I couldn't have a stress echo cardiogram, a set of tests that are carried out while you are actually exercising ie; on a tread mill, because of this damage to my sternum and because of my injured leg

I couldn't have an echogram because I now couldn't lie on my side because of the sternum swelling and due to the size of my chest they always had difficulty examining or should I say imaging my heart.

So for good measure I was also sent for a stress echo and a nuclear profusion test of my heart, this is unbelievably scary stuff.

While still on the ward a young lady turned up with a huge lead apron on and carrying a lead encased box.

Within this box was a lead encased syringe containing radio active liquid which she, once my name had been confirmed, squeezed into my arm and then wandered off.

Ten minutes later a chap turned up with a wheel chair and carter me down to cardiac investigations where I was helped into a scanner, very much like an MRI machine, cylindrical but much smaller, so small in fact that I had to hold my arms above my head while laying flat on my back, the rotating part of the machine still brushed my chest as it passed over me. It took for ever to get me into the machine, I could hardly help with a broken chest but eventually I was in, all I could then think about was how I was going to get out again.

To facilitate the above, a beautiful Asian nurse had to hold or support the weight of my arms throughout the scan, some twenty minutes,

Half way through the scan they inject another liquid by remote control to make the heart work a little harder and measure the differences.

I then, the next day, had a stress echo, similar to the above where you are sat up in a chair and contrast liquids are injected into you which show up when viewed with an ultra sound scanner, your heart is then sped up with another liquid and the muscles can be seen as the heart starts to work harder. During this test, the doctor induced massive Angina in me so had to stop quickly by reversing the drug.

They probably regret sending me on the above missions because it revealed extensive heart damage, enough for my diagnosis to now show as "profound heart failure"

I was kept in bed and on anti biotic tablets, lots of injections and insulin again while the chest infection cleared up and went home on day nine feeling I might add a whole lot better physically but not the least bit happy with what had been found, the chest has now still not joined and will be a permanent feature and one that will deter if not prevent do again by-pass surgery in the future so my prognosis is very bleak.

During this stay I was again confronted with a lunatic, not his fault as usual but this one really took the biscuit.

He had been born rather damaged; his lower limbs hadn't grown so he had the legs of a two year old and the cock of a chaffinch.

Sadly his upper bits had grown and while he had the mind of a dining table he had the mouth of a very big crowd.

He had been left quite a lot of money by his now dead parents and while in hospital had a private full time carer who was terrified of upsetting him, the nutter had already bought the carer a really nice car, partly for running himself around as well as for the carers private use and the nutter was not slow apparently, in telling his carers superiors if he was being unkind to him.

This left the scenario where this chap, who's name was John, could do and say what ever he wanted without fear of retribution and he bloody well did just that.

It all started when he arrived into our unit of the ward one quiet afternoon, he was suffering with an infection in his cock because he was immobile and had to totally rely on his carers to keep him clean and provide him with and fit this little contraption that slid over his tiny little willy which then drained his bladder into the normal bag on the side of the bed

The trouble was, his cock, which was no more than half an inch long couldn't have a catheter up it so he had to have one around it, even so, he shit the bed at least once everyday, into a nappy supposedly, probably out of spite because he couldn't piss the bed with this contraption fitted.

He got off on the wrong foot with me by yelling and shouting his orders to both the intimidated carer and the nursing staff, waking me up from my mid day nap which was important as I didn't sleep well at night.

I was totally pissed off, I am sure that the nursing staff gave me a nutter out of spite for complaining about the big bloke earlier on who wiped shit down my curtains.

As soon as John saw me he started repeatedly saying to me, "hello, whats your name" over and over again and although at first I told him my name he had forgotten it within two minutes and the conversation started all over again.

His carer had taken this opportunity to do a bunk for a couple of hours and John kept on and on at me so I got out of bed and pulled his curtains round him so that he couldn't see me but he yelled so loud that the nurses opened them again and guess what his first question was, you guessed it, hello, whats your name ?

I pulled my curtains around this time but shut up he would not because he still couldn't see me, I am not his problem though, he has become mine.

You may think that I am nasty or mean, I am not normally, I do not enjoy being confronted with this type of person when it does not suit me, ie pushed in my face and I cannot get away and he didn't shut up until I went over to his bed and told him that I was going to cut his throat while he was asleep if he didn't shut up and stay quiet.

The above worked until his carer came back and was told what I had done, I then had to offer the same to the carer, I really wasn't amused and cannot abide jealousy.

Once again, I decided that it was time to go home, if they couldn't keep the sanity at even a basic level I didn't want to play and Linda picked me up, grateful again for not having to visit each day, I do believe the nutters were starting to wear her down as well.

When she arrived to see me, there was always someone who wanted her attention as well, normally first and after a bit it is quite hard to care.

The above correct diagnosis triggered a spate of appointments for me as the John Radcliffe NHS Trust attempted to cover its arse especially after I noted everything that had happened to the trust directors and various heads of chair person and head of departments. Please note, if you were left out and were not complained about I am sure you will fuck up soon and I can add your name then.

I had catalogued all cock ups, all incorrect diagnosis, my nutters and loonies list and especially how bloody minded the cardiac consultant had been when he had told me that everything was ok, he is the best and everything will be ok.

I was offered appointments with pain clinics, rehabilitation consultants, emotional stress consultants, cardio thoracic surgeons, vascular consultants, renal consultants, orthopaedic consultants and anybody else who had an interest or didn't want to be left out inclusive of paediatricians in case I was just being a big baby.

I had letters of apology, letters of appointment and have now been offered a knighthood.

Starting at the beginning of this huge list and this all happened inside one month, I went to see the pain clinic, which, for convenience sake is in a different hospital, hidden away in an old building, miles from where you can park, what pratt worked this one out knowing that I had difficulty with walking.

I saw a professor nobody, and after an examination and a flick through my notes, he had the very abbreviated version, not available on DVD, he told me that it was fine to stop on the MST morphine sulphate and Paracetomol provided I didn't increase the dose, I told him that had already been assumed by my GP and that I was sorry to have wasted my time, not his time I might add.

He did as a closing peace offering suggest immediate pain relief once a week, injections into the sternum and around my neck, if that would help, I advised my aversion to needles and left before he got his witch doctor dolls and prayer beads out of the drawer.

The next on the list was some physio therapists who examined me and advised what exercise I should be doing, none was their best gambit as this was so unusual that neither had training to make a judgement, they offered to have a guess if I promised not to quote them.

It was then the turn of the shrinks, for want of a better word, offering all forms of emotional crutches, normally wrapped up in a brochure or two and even asking would I like to see the hospital pastoral team, even the shrinks in this hospital believe in the almighty.

The cardio thoracic teams and the vascular people were a different kettle of fish because all they did was to try damage limitation, thought I was out for a quick buck or two by suing someone and no matter what we said it was obvious that no one wanted to talk to me and all closed up with the surgeon, professor Taggart adopting the answer," it was all perfect, I am the very best and the job was perfect and you have nothing wrong with you"

We hadn't said it wasn't a perfect piece of surgery, we just knew that something had been going wrong, wasn't right and now wasn't going to improve, we just wanted some answers for what is happening with my life, my job, my family, my future, could I please have a prognosis without you all being scared for your own sakes.

We, Linda and I, learnt nothing more from them and it was to be a long time before we did.

I was then sent to see Mr Green, his name I do remember because I think one should remember another mans name when he messes about with your cock as much as Mr Green messed about with mine.

The procedure to find out why I had no or little feeling down below was humiliating, embarrassing and the most awful thing that has happened to me in my life, worse than the camera up the arse because when they do that you are looking the other way, not looking them all in the face while they mess with your cock.

The procedure needs telling, it is so awful that the whole thing is hilariously funny, I wasn't laughing at the time I might add.

The chap plus two nurses who were on hand for a mix of training, assisting and having a jolly good time got me to strip off and lie on a bed, normal sort of examination bed, cold and far too small for me.

The gentleman gets one of the nurses to hold my willy, with gloves on, and he injects an anaesthetic into my Japs eye, telling me as he does it that it will sting for a while, he is quite right to, it does sting for quite a while but to take my mind off of the stinging he asks me to roll over and rather roughly shoves a probe straight up my arse, leaving wires hanging out, and rolls me back over. I have treated dead turkeys with more consideration and respect.

He then inserts a tube with wires inside of it into my cock and pushes it all the way up to my bladder, if he had pushed it in any further I am sure it would have been sticking out of my nose like a wandering tape worm.

He then, with the help of his admirers, filled my bladder for me using a funnel attached to the end of the pipe that was sticking out of my cock and was held above his head.

And when I was about to explode he asked me to stand up and pee into the container in front of me, while the pipe was still in my cock and the wires were still hanging out of my arse, the pee mostly going on my feet at this time, picture it, if you are sad enough. All of the above took about fifteen or twenty minutes and I do not recommend it, unless it is part of a TV game show.

From the above saga he was able to deduce that I have very poor flow and no electric nerve activity to my bladder, ie my brain had stopped communicating with my bladder, prostate or sphincter, this I could understand, why would my brain want to talk to my arsehole ?

He asked me to get dressed, after he had painfully removed my pipes and wires and we all sat down in a little huddle for a chat where the topic of conversation was my cock and its loneliness.

He advised that the computer, yes the wires were actually attached to something, the computer and data told him that I had had a stroke, a mini one admittedly but a stroke all the same and in all probability this would not improve, I was stuck with a semi dead cock.

I picked up my dignity and left wondering what the hell had just happened to me and asking myself why a grown man would want to do that for a living, I also vowed never ever to put myself through it again because the embarrassment of the above event had made my cock so scared that it did its best to hide and for those few minutes I had the smallest cock in the world.

How on earth had I managed to have so many children.

I am now at the London University College Hospital, I have elected to come here for two reasons.

One is that I go past the doors everyday on my way into and out of London and the second being that it was showing the lowest infection rates within a given radius from home and as I had caught an infection with my last four surgical procedures I decided this to be a good starting point. As a side venture, my doctor was very pleased to be able to send me here because she had qualified at this teaching hospital.

I am to be seen by yet another Indian doctor who is examining my right ankle which has been badly sprained five times until it eventually broke and had to be pinned back together, an infection during its mending period has left it both painful and unreliable, I have a habit of falling over, which was why it was pinned in the first place...

The idea is, in conjunction with my knee repairs, that I will be able to get regular exercise if they get on and do the surgery, something that none of them seem willing to undertake given the risk with my rather sad heart condition, or lack of condition.

This chap, obviously primed by the oxford hospital, agrees to do the surgery but even a year later I have yet to get my appointment.

I have also been seen by another chap who is going to replace my knees, and again much later and I am still waiting, limping and not walking too well.

Chapter twelve

It is March 2008 now and I am back in the hospital cardiac day care unit where I am going to have an angio gram again, the first one since being in High Wycombe hospital all that time ago, strangely I am feeling rather anxious about it.

I have been trying to live a normal life, decorating, gardening even working three days a week but it is obvious now that my breathing has become very laboured with any exertion at all and the occasional tumble, or collapse shows that I really am not at all well.

My GP has been annoying the JR staff, calling and writing until she gets a result, normally pushing me up waiting lists and together we have tackled the Trust directors who while not admitting to anything are trying to get me seen to quicker if only to stop my letters and my doctors telephone calls.

We are not being unreasonable, this is after all unfinished business, it would compare to priming your car to stop it rusting but not getting on with applying the finish coats.

I have become well known to two of the consultant cardiologists Mr Oliver Ormerod and Dr Bernard Prendergast who are extremely clever and professional doctors who obviously specialise in treatment without cutting your chest open first.

Dr Prendergast is the first to put some stents into me, a stent being a small cylindrical tube of gauze, metal and normally coated with a slow release drug to stop or prevent you rejecting it, which would prove fatal.

They are normally between 3 and 5mm thick and 10-20mm in length, and following a shave and an incision in the groin or wrist, they are slid up your artery to where the blockage is at the heart muscle and then blown up and locked into place with a small balloon, the balloon being removed, all quite painless and fairly quick with only an hour or so per session, no stitches and normally home the same day.

I had two of these stents fitted to my by-pass grafts which were all now showing some measure of blockage or narrowing and immediately felt an improvement in my breathing, obviously due to the sudden increase in blood flowing to my starved heart muscle, cheers all round because this indicated a treatment could be made to work.

After a plug is fitted to the wound I was wheeled back to the ward and Dr Prendergast popped in to tell me the good and the bad news, the bad being now obvious to me in that the open heart surgery by-pass grafting had not worked and had all blocked up, the good news being that the stents appeared to work and I was showing an immediate improvement which was very encouraging.

This has taken two minutes to write down and two minutes for you to read it but that really doesn't do it all justice, it really is the most incredible adventure, having someone work on your heart remotely with you wide awake and on the whole, pain free.

I went home that same night, walking like I had been kicked in the bollocks but walking none the less.

I did feel better and was able to do so much more now, I could even walk better because I didn't get the dead feeling it my legs which was caused, I am led to believe, by circulation problems, my legs filling up with blood.

I was able to work a bit more and generally enjoy myself, taking my children swimming etc, I hadn't booked up for the marathon though, I was still quite poorly and my diabetes was playing me up more and more and it seemed as though each time they did something to my heart I would need my diabetes medicines adjusting or couldn't control my sugar levels with the occasional Hypo, passing out in a public place being a really good way to get attention.

This happened one Saturday when I didn't have any breakfast and took the children for a swim, running out of sugar while in the pool and collapsing half way through a hand stand, while still in the pool I might add, scaring the daylights out of the kids and ending up with another ride in the ambulance. Sorry Hannah.

I have now come to understand the signs now a bit better, I can feel the start of a sweat which means I need food, sugar, carbs or even just a simple banana and I very rarely test my blood these days.

It seems to have taken me ages to get used to being a diabetic, I do not generally like breakfast for at least a couple of hours after I am out of bed and this is still causing me problems if I leave the house and don't find somewhere to stop and eat.

Things plod on up to autumn of 2008 when I am poorly again and this time it is Oliver Ormerod who carries out the surgery, this time two other grafts are subjected to the unblocking, expanding and fitting of stents, all going well and home next day this time, more tests needed before I could go home same day.

This time the screens are set at such an angle that I can see what is going on, I can see the large mammary graft, where a large piece of my leg artery rather than just a piece of vein, has been grafted high up in my chest behind the mammary muscles, pectoral muscles if you want and I can see it all the way down to my heart.

In the middle of its length it is pinched closed, as though you were pinching a drinking straw in the middle until it was shut.

I can see the balloon which is being used to open up the blockage, going into place and I feel the Angina coming on really strong now as the blood flowing to my heart is restricted further while they work on it.

I have to make my self lie very still and breath in slow motion while they slide the stent into place and then again while they blow it up to fix it, they cant ever be taken out again and are worth more than £1000.00 each without the cost of the technicians, surgeons and hire of the lab not least the cost of a day in hospital, once again I feel much better when the stent is in place with noticeable breathing improvement.

For good measure another stent is fitted to the forth by-pass graft so in theory they are all partly unblocked though that clearly isn't the case, I still have very restricted flow and a stress echo shows heart muscle damage and very bad flow still on one side of my heart.

The staff in the day care unit all know of me by name now as do the consultants and surgeons, I am not sure if this is a good thing or bad.

Are they keen to help me or are they in dread of being the one who cocks it up or had me die on the table with a lot of explaining to do and messy paperwork, I am definitely visiting far too often but really do need the work done and each time they find and unblock a bit more I really do feel the benefit.

I have been up to York to see my middle son Thomas, he is home with a badly twisted ankle and needed to go to the hospital for a check up and replacement cast, as I was sat around and I had nothing better to do I popped up and took him there, it sounds a long way from oxford but on average only takes between three and four hours each way.

His fiancée, Rachael, made me welcome and went off to work leaving us to play on the computer and games console, we were yelling with laughter, always a good medicine.

We had an absolutely fantastic time doing this, I do not remember the last time that I laughed so much and suffered for my pains, nearly had death by X box which would have been interesting reading especially for the younger generation who would have loved it on my grave.

The game, when played on a high definition very large screen television is so realistic that when someone steps round a corner to shoot or stab you, you jump with fear and in my case, my heart is going bonkers and I quickly get feelings of palpitation etc.

Tom makes me stop playing before I kick the bucket but we really do enjoy playing these games, Death by Xbox, how cool would that is.

Dr Prendergast has just got me into the day unit really quickly and fitted a stent within a stent, quite an unusual practice and he is shocked that all four grafts and now all four stents are badly blocked or narrowed, he knows not why this is happening, quite unusual he tells me.

Managed to get in and out in a single day but this leaves me with big questions and my Dr,s and consultants with no answers for me.

Apparently the above is quite unheard of and very unusual, no one knows why I am blocking up, it is though I am trying to reject the stents now.

It is November 2008 and I am not getting any better, in fact I am getting quickly much worse, I have lost all muscle in my arms and legs as well as my back and stomach which leaves me as a big bag of fat especially as I am the same weight as before, nearly twenty four stones.

I can hardly walk anymore because of my very bad ankle and sore knees, I hardly ever ride my beautiful motor bike anymore even though we have had some fabulous weather, by the time I have bent down and taken off the covers and locks I am already knackered and sweating, as soon as I have covered ten miles or so my arms are aching with Angina and my knees start to hurt, a lot, so I may as well sell my bike now.

It is getting impossible to continue, I cannot work, the business has failed and will be with the receiver in a couple of weeks, I cannot swim, walk or have any fun without getting breathless and in pain, even simple gardening has become beyond me.

I haven't had sex for over two years now, the last attempt lasted about fifteen seconds before I needed an ambulance, which was a very interesting conversation with the hospital when asked what I was doing. In actual fact I was quite impressed with the fifteen seconds.

I feel guilty and embarrassed for being lazy, I sit down while Linda is still charging around doing things, I sit because I have to but it doesn't stop me from wishing otherwise.

I stay around for Linda and the children, I would like to dose myself up with pain killers and ride across to the continent on my motor bike with a few grand in my pocket and find somewhere nice to sit down and die, as I type this I have waves of pain cascading across my chest and through my back, life has become a miserable burden and I think daily of committing the ultimate sin and pack it all in, let it go, give in.

Dr Prendergast has had a good look at my bollocks again, he never looks me in the eye, always got his head next to my bollock.s

As I am so considerate, I have had tattooed on my scrotum the words, "caution, may contain nuts",

It is 13th April 2009 and I am back in the catheter lab having another Angio gram, this is becoming a filthy habit, having my groin shaved so often and putting my tackle on display.

Sadly I have been left very late in the day and haven't eaten now for some eighteen hours and I am really feeling very rough, can really feel the diabetes getting out of control.

I have spent the previous few hours letting the staff know that I haven't eaten, I am diabetic and I am about to have a Hypo ie; I am running out of sugar and need to eat, deaf ears though and I am still sent to the lab even though it is nearing tea time.

By the time I get to theatre, I have walked down with an attendant nurse, I am clearly in trouble and having a Hypo, had to sit down and I am starting to sweat up badly, nausier washing over me like the tide on a beach.

The technicians try to carry on with the procedure, I have a limited slot booked and do not want to miss it, they strip me off and lay me down, wash and shave me, and get started, I have the smoothest set of balls in the whole world because they are forever being washed and shaved though I am not so sure about the skin down there, it feels hard and lumpy, probably all of the bits and bobs they keep shoving in.

No sooner had the technician got the catheter into the incision that I start to feel really poorly and they start shooting me with anti sickness drugs and get me some Lucazade to drink, sadly it stayed down but a few minutes before I began showing them what an Olympic class vomitter can do, I chucked it everywhere, I was being held down at this point because the man by my balls was yelling at me to stay still due to the wire still in my heart and the catheter in my groin so I had to twist only my shoulders and my neck round so as to vomit into or try and vomit into a dish, my shoulders do not twist round due to my broken chest so that was even more fun, picture it if you will….if your sad.

Great big fat bloke, naked on an operating table with shaven bollocks and pipes sticking out of his groin being held down while he is soaked in sweat from head to foot, projectile vomiting in a operating theatre or lab with six nurses trying to hold him down while other people are trying to insert needles into his arms, all the while the fat bloke praying to his God to let him die.

That is exactly how it was, they had to get the wire and catheter out and plug the hole in my groin, cancel the procedure and clean me and everything up, they should have listened to me.

They got me to the ward but I was by now to poorly to go home so was admitted to the general cardiac ward, I was cleaned up some more and put on a glucose drip to get my sugar level back up.

I couldn't even get my willy into a bottle to take a pee, the nurse had to do that for me, the willy bit, not take a pee for me, but this nurse remembers me from previous visits and I remember her Rachael, ward staff nurse.

I am violently sick all night and can't eat or drink, can't keep food down so stay on Glucose drips until morning when things seem to settle down and I stop feeling quite so ill, providing I do not attempt to move.

Obviously Dr Prendergast is rather concerned about yesterdays cock up and pays me a visit mid afternoon where he advises that I didn't just have a Hypo, he feels I had a mini stroke but should be ok in a few days and that I could go home that same evening.

I couldn't walk too well as I was completely dizzy and Linda, bless her, had to push me in a wheel chair, not for the first time I might add, all the way to the exit, I think she hurt her back doing it. I did frequently ask her to stop and let me walk but she wouldn't hear of it, I don't think I could have walked out of the hospital anyway and she left me in the reception area at the front of the hospital while she recovered the car and drove it round to collect me.

I am two and a half times her weight and with the bags and things she was pushing at least three times her own weight but she would not let me try and walk in case I fell over and we couldn't go home. We both feel somewhat let down by the system here, once discharged from the ward it would appear that all responsibility for you is lifted and you have to make your own way out and away, a bit stiff really, no nurses and doctors gathered around the entrance waving you off, wishing you well, like in the hospital programs.

In the hospital programs people are sitting up having a cup of tea twenty minutes after heart surgery, I wish they would get real.

Linda got up with me this morning at 04.45 so that I could go into London for a meeting, I was too ill to go on my own and although I did manage to drive there and back it was good to know that I had some back up. We have to get up really early because it takes such a long time for her to do her bloody hair.

The meeting was very important and could not be re scheduled, in the end it was all a waste of time because we still haven't been paid what is due and was promised so the business will fold anyway, in some ways not a bad thing because it is far too much of a struggle for me to keep it all going now.

Linda got a good quality fried breakfast out of it as well which has shown her that not all builders eat rubbish fatty breakfasts, the café at the end of the road from the site does a lovely clean plate of food.

I can drive but am too dizzy to walk unaided, still have some nausea to deal with but generally I am on the mend, I think.

I had been to see the receiver today and put the business into administration, very worried as I do not see how some of the debts will not bounce back to bite me and I am worried about not having any income, I am after all completely unemployable, far to high a risk for anyone to employ.

I think the worry and anxiety is going to be what keeps me feeling so poorly all of the time, I can feel pains building up when the telephone rings or there is a knock on the door, feel my blood pressure going up and down like a yoyo, not good at all.

I have been to see my doctor, we collectively agree that I have developed another ulcer from all of the stress and worry.

She changes come of my drugs, reduces my blood pressure control drug because this is what she feels could be making me dizzy when I stand up and increases my ulcer drugs, I start to feel better within a couple of days, bless her.

I quite quickly get another appointment come through for Dr Prendergast to complete what he started and aborted last month, though my groin is still rather tender and my bollock stubble rather short.

Normally you are supposed to wait three months between procedures to give things a chance to settle down and let the plug in the artery melt away but he obviously knows what he is doing.

Having had such a cock up last time I am going to the lab mid morning, before I get hungry and I have given myself a shot of morphine to help.

I am washed and shaved as usual and injected in the area of incision with anaesthetic, a hole is made and they are in, really off like a rocket today as I think they want to get the maximum usage of what time we have. I am pleased to see Dr Prendergast again so soon, he is a nice chap, a smiling honest looking face which helps alleviate some of the anxiety.

Dr Prendergast quickly finds the area that he has been looking for, a major blockage in one of my by-pass grafts and inserts a stent, all seems to be going well then.

Just when I think it is time to finish, I am feeling quite good so there is no rush from my point of view, the team has a little chat about what they can see and decide to have another bash with a second stent.

I am by now feeling very sore in my groin and have been lying still on my back for an hour already but Dr Prendergast feels it prudent to maximise the repairs with this additional work, my seventh stent, my heart will be worth a kings ransom if I could give the stents up, sadly I cannot.

This second stent of the day takes a good deal of work, pushing and shoving, balloons in and out but eventually agreement is reached by the technicians that a good result has been achieved, the stent is in situ with the first one making a continuous opening and although I am very sore I feel that my breathing has improved.

I am taken back to the ward, have a sandwich and a cup of tea and have to lie still for four hours with the hourly inspections of my groin, all looks to be ok and I was able to go home that evening at six o'clock, my usual driver in attendance.

Just before we departed, Dr Prendergast popped in to see me and added "you have had more than an entire years worth of x-ray radiation, your chest may burn and your skin may go red but nothing really to worry about", we thanked him for not worrying us and left.

I was feeling very very sore in my chest, Dr Prendergast had already told me that it had been difficult to get the second stent into place and that my heart would have suffered some bruising and my groin was very alive.

That same day I collapsed in the bathroom after feeling terrible chest pain during the night, it was so bad that I thought that I was having a heart attack, couldn't stay conscious and Linda called the ambulance again, the nine number on our telephone has worn off, it has had so much use.

Usual route, fire engine, ambulance, blues and twos to the JR and after some morphine and into bed, ECG and bloods taken for testing to see if I had had another episode.

I stayed the night and through the next day until all had settled down again, the pain going away, and then sent home and off to my own bed as I was still rough. Again, it was thought to just be the extremes of so much surgery, so many intrusions to my heart that it has just had enough, my chest hurts so much nearly all of the time that a good breath in is beyond me, I shallow breath now as a habit and a yawn or cough are major events with extensive pain.

The saga goes on, I have had a heart attack, a quadruple heart by-pass, a stroke followed by a coma, seven stents have been fitted in the by-pass grafts during which I suffered another minor stroke and my chest bones have refused to join.

I have heart failure and still cannot walk very well nor climb any stairs so in reality, I have become a cripple for the sake of staying alive......... Is this really being alive?

At the very least I can take comfort in the knowledge that what I am going through will help the next generation, the cock ups that I have been through will add to the ocean of knowledge and make things easier for those who follow, we hope......

My eldest son has today had a stent fitted, he is twenty nine years old.

My middle son still smokes even though he is fully aware of the consequences, he is twenty seven years old

My youngest son carries too much weight and does little or no exercise, he is off to the doctors for a check up, he is fifteen...

It really is a family curse after all....................................

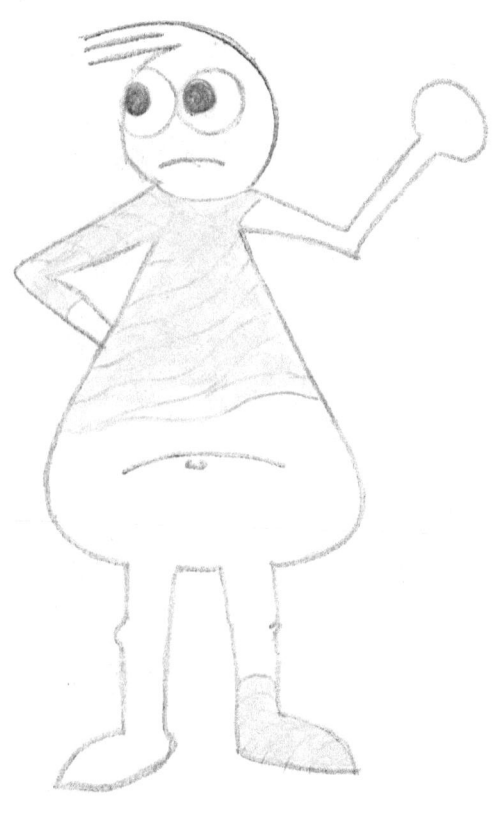